DATE DUE

MAR 1 5 1994	NOV 1 4 2000
OCT - 5 1994	MAR 5 2001
	FEB 1 2002
NOV 1 2 1994	APR 1 8 2002
MAR 2 6 1995	
APR 1 0 1995	
OCT 2 3 1995	
NOV - 2 1995	
FEB 2 3 1996	
OCT 2 2 1997	
NOV 0 6 1997	
NOV 1 5 1997	
NOV 2 0 1997	
FEB 0 9 1999	
MAR 1 8 1999	
MAR 3 0 1999	

Postpartum
Depression

Clinical Nursing Research Series

The purpose of this series, **Clinical Nursing Research**, is to provide a concise description of the research on specific issues in nursing that are relevant to the practitioner. Authors report their own research findings and examine other important research in that area, paying close attention to the implications for practice and specifically addressing intervention techniques. The series will inform the nurse researcher of some of the significant research being conducted and help practicing nurses enhance their expertise.

In this series . . .

Postpartum Depression: A Comprehensive Approach for Nurses
by Kathleen A. Kendall-Tackett, with Glenda Kaufman Kantor

Alzheimer's Disease and Marriage
by Lore K. Wright

Postpartum Depression

A Comprehensive Approach for Nurses

Kathleen A. Kendall-Tackett
with Glenda Kaufman Kantor

Sage Series in Clinical Nursing Research

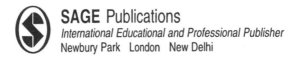

SAGE Publications
International Educational and Professional Publisher
Newbury Park   London   New Delhi

Copyright © 1993 by Sage Publications, Inc.

For information address:

SAGE Publications, Inc.
2455 Teller Road
Newbury Park, California 91320

SAGE Publications Ltd.
6 Bonhill Street
London EC2A 4PU
United Kingdom

SAGE Publications India Pvt. Ltd.
M-32 Market
Greater Kailash I
New Delhi 110 048 India

Printed in the United States of America

Library of Congress Cataloging-in-Publication Data

Kendall-Tackett, Kathleen A.
　　Postpartum depression: a comprehensive approach for nurses /
Kathleen A. Kendall-Tackett, Glenda Kaufman Kantor.
　　　　p.　　cm.—(Clinical nursing research)
　　Includes bibliographical references and index.
　　ISBN 0-8039-5034-9 (cl).—ISBN 0-8039-5035-7 (pb)
　　　　1. Postpartum depression.　2. Postpartum depression—Nursing.
I. Kantor, Glenda Kaufman.　II. Title.　III. Series: Clinical
nursing research (Unnumbered)
　　　[DNLM: 1. Depression—nurses' instruction.　2. Depressive
disorders—nurses' instruction.　3. Psychotic disorders—nurses'
instruction.　4. Pueperal disorders—nurses' instruction.　WM 171 K33]
RG852.K45　1993
618.7'6—dc20
DNLM/DLC　　　　　　　　　　　　　　　　　　　　　　92-48669

93　94　95　96　10　9　8　7　6　5　4　3　2　1

Sage Production Editor:　Diane S. Foster

To my sons, Kenneth and Christopher, who have enriched my life and provided the best possible education on the postpartum period.

Contents

Preface

The birth of a baby is a profound and life-changing event. As with other life transitions, the passage can be stressful. After giving birth, a woman may experience many feelings, ranging from joy to deep sadness and depression. According to Sears (1991), approximately 100,000 North American women are treated for postpartum depression each year, with an estimated 4,000 being so severely affected that they must be hospitalized. And these figures may represent only the tip of the iceberg. With so many suffering from postpartum illness, it is truly surprising that so few clinical texts dedicate more than a few pages to it, if indeed they mention it at all.

Authors of popular books on postpartum depression often lament over the lack of information available and conclude that no one is interested in this topic. Information is available, however, and many studies have been conducted on postpartum depression. Unfortunately the results of this research are often difficult to find. Studies on postpartum depression appear in a dizzying array of journals, authored by researchers in such diverse fields as nursing, psychology, psychiatry, cognitive science, pediatrics, and, to a lesser extent, obstetrics. The purpose of this book is to make this information accessible to clinicians who work with new mothers.

My decision to write this book for nurses was an easy one. In my 9 years as a child abuse researcher, I have seen for myself the vital and often heroic role that nurses play in working with young families. This book was written especially for nurses who work directly with new mothers on maternity units or NICU's, in obstetricians' and pediatricians' offices, as childbirth educators, as visiting nurses, as nurse practitioners, or as nurse-midwives. To write for a nursing audience, I enlisted the aid of my friend and colleague Glenda Kaufman Kantor. She brings to this project a formidable background, having been an obstetrical and neonatal nurse, professor of nursing, childbirth educator, lactation consultant, and nurse practitioner in gynecology. She is also a sociologist and full-time researcher and thus provides both clinical and research perspectives.

In this book Glenda and I have integrated the findings of empirical research. We organized this book around the assumption that the causes of postpartum illness are heterogeneous and that there can be multiple causes for depression within the same woman. Postpartum depression may be due to a combination of biological, psychological, and social factors, and several studies have examined multiple possible causes (Affonso & Arizmendi, 1986; Cutrona, 1983; O'Hara, Neunaber, & Zekoski, 1984; O'Hara, Schlechte, Lewis, & Varner, 1991). This multicausal model is analogous to a risk-factor approach to heart disease. Although not everyone who smokes, is obese, or has high blood cholesterol levels, high blood pressure, or a sedentary life-style develops heart disease, these factors increase an individual's risk. Further, the more of these factors present, the greater the risk. For this book we expand even further on previous research by including all the major risk factors that have been identified. Our goal is to describe the whole range of factors that might put women at increased risk for developing postpartum depression.

For the book to have scientific integrity, Glenda and I have not attempted to gloss over areas where the state of knowledge in the field is limited. Rather we have attempted to provide you with enough information about studies so that you can form your own opinions. In some cases the most definitive answer that we can give is "it depends." Throughout this book we have included the stories of 22 women who have experienced either postpartum depression or psychosis. These women were recruited from an advertisement in the national newsletter of Depression After Delivery (one woman was recruited from a

NICU support group). Seventeen of these women were interviewed by telephone through the use of an open-ended interview that typically lasted an hour to an hour and a half. The other five women chose to share their stories in writing. They ranged in age from 25-39 years, and most had experienced their depressions or psychoses within the past 2 years. They represented 16 different states and one Canadian province.

The first chapter focuses on definitions and symptoms of postpartum depression. Infanticide, maternal suicide, and obsessional thoughts about harming the baby are also described. Chapter 2 focuses on physiological factors, including hormones, postpartum pain, and fatigue. The risks and benefits of antidepressant medications are also described. Chapter 3 focuses on negative birth experiences, including a conceptual model of aspects of birth that can make the experience traumatic, the processing of traumatic events, and a detailed discussion on the psychological ramifications of cesarean birth.

Chapter 4 describes psychosocial causes of postpartum illness. The psychological factors include the mother's way of looking at the world (her attributional style), how competent she feels as a parent, and her previous psychiatric history. The social causes include the effect of negative life events, and the buffering influence of social support. Chapter 5 describes the infant's role in postpartum depression, specifically focusing on how infant temperament or illness affects the mother-infant relationship. Chapter 6 is an in-depth examination of one woman's story of postpartum depression and psychosis. In Chapter 7 final suggestions are made and a plan for prevention that can be used by individual mothers is presented.

At the end of each chapter, specific suggestions for intervention are offered that involve identifying the problem, educating new mothers, and providing referrals to appropriate community resources. These suggestions are meant to offer something to nurses in many types of professional settings, and not every suggestion may be helpful for you. The goal is to provide the widest possible range of alternatives. The first chapter provides an overview of postpartum depression.

KATHLEEN A. KENDALL-TACKETT

Acknowledgments

This book would not have been possible without the assistance of many people. We would like to thank the nurses who graciously offered to review this manuscript and provide feedback: Janis Tuxbury, R.N.; Michelle Gilliland, R.N.; Patsy Kling, R.N.; and Joanne Emerick, B.S.N.

Preparation of this manuscript was funded by NIMH grant T32 MH15161 to the first author. We would like to thank the staff of the Family Research Laboratory at the University of New Hampshire for their assistance during every phase of this project, and the members of the Family Research Laboratory's seminar group for their helpful comments and suggestions. We are indebted to Ying Peng, Tina Colacchio, and Dan Bourgain for their careful library research, and to Patricia VanWagoner for her thoughtful editorial assistance.

The national office of Depression After Delivery provided a great deal of assistance, both in helping us locate women who were willing to share their stories and in providing background information and materials. The women whom we interviewed have added immeasurably to this book. We are grateful for their willingness to share their experiences with us, even though this was sometimes painful. We admire them for their courage, honesty, and willingness to help others.

We are grateful to Christine Smedley at Sage Publications for supporting this project from the beginning and for providing many helpful suggestions along the way. We also appreciate the thoughtful feedback of an anonymous reviewer, whose comments improved our manuscript.

Finally, many thanks to Doug Tackett. He made this project possible and enthusiastically supported it through each phase.

ONE

An Overview of
Postpartum Depression

In the hospital, everything was wonderful. . . . People visited me, bringing gifts and telling me how darling my son was. I was on a high. But 5 days later I sat at home, rocking my baby, tears streaming down my face, thinking "I can't do this job. I absolutely can't handle all this responsibility." (Moore, 1990, p. 34)

Motherhood. The word conjures up such attractive images. The perfectly coiffed young woman holding her angelic sleeping baby. Her house is spotless, her handsome and adoring husband is nearby. As attractive as this image is, however, it is far from the reality that many new mothers face. Some women find their transition to motherhood less than smooth. They may feel overwhelmed, isolated, and depressed—even at the point when they seem to have everything they could possibly want (Oakley, 1983). They may be suffering from postpartum depression.

Postpartum depression is a condition that can isolate women at a time when they most need the help of others. They may be ashamed to admit that life with a new baby is not always bliss. They may assume that everyone else has made a smoother transition to motherhood than they have. And they may be truly embarrassed that they are not able to cope better (Dix, 1985; Kitzinger, 1975). Melissa, who suffered from depression after both of her children were born, describes her sense of embarrassment:

AUTHORS' NOTE: Some names have been changed.

In my [childbirth education] class, they mentioned the baby blues and told us if it goes beyond "normal," to contact them. I didn't know what normal was. I was shocked when I found out [later] how mild the baby blues were. What people experienced as the baby blues, I was experiencing a year later. I went back later and told them to provide more information in their classes. . . . With the first child, there was such a feeling of shame. I thought every woman went through this, and I couldn't handle it.

Unfortunately, professionals can contribute to women's shame and embarrassment by minimizing their symptoms or by attempting to convince them that what they are experiencing is "normal." Debbie, who suffered from depression after the birth of each of her four children, describes how other people tended to minimize the seriousness of her depression every time she experienced it.

I think my depression was obvious to the nurses. Not one of them even recognized it or asked if they could help. Health care people don't realize that it has an effect on people. They just brush it aside and say the "blues" will ease up. These were *not* the blues. . . . I went to my OB and told him about my depression. I went to him after each pregnancy. He always said, "It must be something else. You're worrying too much about this." He sent me to a counselor after the first pregnancy. I saw her for 3 weeks. She thought I needed stimulation and to go back to work. I did go back to work, and it helped somewhat, but I knew that was not the root of my depression. Consequently I refused to seek help from counselors after my second and third pregnancies. [She sought help after her fourth child was born.]

As we shall demonstrate in later sections of this book, postpartum depression can have serious consequences, especially if left untreated (McGrath, Keita, Strickland, & Russo, 1990). Its symptoms should never be ignored or minimized, as it can wreak havoc on entire families (Kitzinger, 1975). The longest lasting effects may be on the children. These effects include lower IQ scores (Cogill, Caplan, Alexandra, Robson, & Kumar, 1986); increased emotional, cognitive, and social problems (O'Hara, 1987); and increased levels of behavioral disturbance at ages 2 months (Whiffen & Gotlib, 1989) and 3 years (Wrate, Rooney, Thomas, & Cox, 1985). In the most serious cases, women will take their own lives or those of their babies (Davidson & Robertson, 1985).

When women become mothers, they are heavily involved in the health care system—both for themselves and for their new babies. Because of this involvement, health care professionals are in key positions to intervene with women suffering from postpartum depression. Nurses in particular are likely to have contact with women who would never seek the services of mental health professionals. Understanding postpartum illness and knowing what signs to look for are vital to any effective intervention. Because many women are reluctant to talk about how they are feeling, you might have to take the first step. The purpose of this book is to better equip you to identify postpartum depression and effectively intervene.

> I believe had the nurses and/or physicians been more "tuned in to" me, they could have helped. . . . I never realized how depressed I was. . . . I was 4 months pregnant with my second child and had no feeling for the new baby to be. I had decided to buy a gun. Fortunately the gun store owner called my husband and inquired as to whether he knew I was purchasing a gun.
>
> Finding help was very difficult. The first psychiatrist found my case "interesting" and wanted to "try" to treat it. I ended up in the hospital OD'd on prescription drugs. Not suicide, but too strong a dose of medication [Kelly].

In the next section, we examine the definitions and symptoms of postpartum illness.

THE THREE FACES
OF POSTPARTUM DEPRESSION

Postpartum depression is a general term that describes three types of illness. These vary in timing of onset, length of episode, and severity of symptoms. The three conditions are (a) postpartum blues, (b) postpartum depression, and (c) postpartum psychosis (Chalmers & Chalmers, 1986; Hopkins, Marcus, & Campbell, 1984; O'Hara, 1987; Stern & Kruckman, 1983; Thirkettle & Knight, 1985). We examine these three types of illness and discuss their relationship to each other.

When defining postpartum depression, professionals frequently raise the question of whether it is distinct from nonpuerperal mental illness. By and large the mental health community acts as if it is not. Some have argued that puerperal and nonpuerperal mental illnesses are similar in terms of their symptomatology and factors predicting onset (O'Hara, 1987) and that the only distinguishing characteristic of puerperal mental illness is an onset associated with childbirth. Further, at the present time no specific diagnostic category for postpartum illness appears in either the *International Classification of Diseases* (ICD-9) or the *Diagnostic and Statistical Manual* (DSM).

In contrast, Dalton (1971) has long argued that postpartum depression is *by definition* specific to the puerperium because it is caused by the sharp drop in progesterone. Therefore it is distinct from nonpostpartum depressions. Chalmers and Chalmers (1986) also argued that postpartum depression is distinct from other depressions. In their view childbirth constitutes a specific stressor that causes depression in an already vulnerable woman. Future research may reveal that the symptoms of postpartum and other depressions are similar but that the puerperium is a time of unique stress. The blues, depression, and psychosis are each described below.

The Blues

> One day I wept and wept, I just couldn't stop, I prayed that nobody would come and visit me, because I don't know how I would have coped. . . . I was just surprised at how weepy I was, because I'm not the kind of person that gets depressed. Mind you, I wasn't really actually depressed. I just felt terribly, terribly worried about the baby and I just couldn't stop crying, you know, for a whole day . . . that was about the fifth day. . . . The next day I was as right as rain again. (Oakley, 1980, p. 115)

"The blues" are commonly described as the weeping and emotional lability that starts shortly after childbirth and lasts only a few days (Leathe, 1987; Snaith, 1983; Stern & Kruckman, 1983). Others have referred to this condition as *depressed mood* (Wrate et al., 1985), *depressive symptoms*[1] (O'Hara, Neunaber, & Zekoski, 1984), or *transient postpartum depression* (Thirkettle &

TABLE 1.1 The Blues: Timing of Onset, Symptoms, and Incidence

Topic	Major findings	References
Onset	3-5 days postpartum typically	Kendell, McGuire, Connor, & Cox (1981); Pitt (1968); Snaith (1983)
Duration	A few days	Kendell, McGuire, Connor, & Cox (1981)
Symptoms	Lability of mood; tearfulness; cognitive confusion; forgetfulness; headaches; depersonalization; negative feelings toward baby; restlessness; irritability; nightmares	Snaith (1983); Thirkettle & Knight (1985)
Incidence	30%-84%, Mean incidence across studies – 55.75%	Thirkettle & Knight (1985) review of the literature

Knight, 1985) to distinguish it from the more serious condition of postpartum depression. "The blues" remains the most common name for this condition, however. A description of symptoms and incidence of the blues is found on Table 1.1.

Although the term *blues* suggests an equivalence with depression or sadness, for many women the crying, lability, anxiety, and confusion may be the most prominent aspects (O'Hara, 1987). A cluster analysis of questionnaire results on postpartum emotional reactions confirmed this notion. Kennerley and Gath (1986) identified seven items that appeared in the cluster they entitled "primary blues": tearful, tired, anxious, overemotional, up and down in mood, low spirited, and muddled in thinking. "Depression" appeared in another cluster.

Until quite recently the blues largely had been overlooked by researchers. Yalom, Lunde, Moos, and Hamburg (1968) noted that because of the ubiquitous nature of the blues, they were not worthy of serious study. Others pointed out, however, that presence of the blues serves as an important barometer of the success of antenatal preparation of the mother or of the medical procedures involved in her care (Thirkettle & Knight, 1985). The blues are also of interest because they represent an opportunity to explore the relationship between mood and biological events and because the blues may predict later postpartum depressions or problems in child management (Hapgood, Elkind, & Wright, 1988; Thirkettle & Knight, 1985).

Postpartum Depression

> The depression started hitting 2 weeks after birth. It really hit hard 2 weeks later [4 weeks postpartum] after cold-turkey weaning. . . . During my depression I escaped from the earth. I am very sociable normally, but I became withdrawn. All my roles changed. My role as a wife, friend, mother, lover, daughter. Even now, I'll never be the same. . . . When I was depressed, I wouldn't do my hair or makeup. I was pale with a poor complexion, and very "drawn" looking. People told me I looked like two different people—like a "before and after" Merle Norman ad [Michelle].

Postpartum depression is a more serious condition than the blues, and the depressive symptoms last longer and are more severe. Information on symptoms and incidence is summarized in Table 1.2. Note that many of the symptoms are similar to those of the blues. This condition is more insidious and can be debilitating (Bridge, Little, Hayworth, Dewhurst, & Priest, 1985; Chalmers & Chalmers, 1986). Joanne describes how her depression affected her. In her case the first symptoms appeared soon after delivery, but the most severe depression occurred at 3 months postpartum.

> Immediately after delivery of my third child, I had a sense of foreboding and anxiety. Since I hadn't slept well after the second baby, I asked for something to help me sleep at night in the hospital. I brought Seconal home from the hospital, but my doctor only gave me 12. That added to the tension. I had difficulty sleeping and very sad hopeless days from the beginning. . . . At 3 months postpartum, there were several nights when I didn't sleep at all. I had anxiety, inability to eat or to nurse—no let down—and very sad, hopeless feelings. . . . I was having an emotional hemorrhage, crying all the time. I was convinced it was my own poor style of living life that caused it. I had no concept that it could be hormonal. . . . It was really shocking what I was experiencing.

Silvia also experienced a variety of symptoms, most prominent among them was anxiety. Her doctors tried several different

TABLE 1.2 Postpartum Depression: Timing of Onset, Symptoms, and Incidence

Topic	Major findings	References
Onset	Within first postpartum year	Bridge, Little, Hayworth, Dewhurst, & Priest (1985)
Duration	At least 2 weeks, but usually longer	Bridge, Little, Hayworth, Dewhurst, & Priest (1985); Chalmers & Chalmers (1986)
Symptoms	Tearfulness; despondency; feelings of inadequacy; numbness; suicidal ideation; sadness; reduced appetite and interest; insomnia; over-sensitivity; feelings of helplessness and hopelessness; excessive dependency; anxiety and despair; irrational fears about baby or mother's health	Affonso & Arizmendi (1986); Chalmers & Chalmers (1986); O'Hara (1987)
Incidence	27% had depressive symptoms at 3-5 months postpartum	Kendell, McGuire, Connor, & Cox (1981); $N = 81$
	20% mild and 8% severe depression at 6 weeks postpartum; 40% mild and 17% severe depression at 12 months postpartum	Bridge, Little, Hayworth, Dewhurst, & Priest (1985); $N = 161$
	12% major and minor depression combined, 9 weeks postpartum	O'Hara, Neunaber, & Zekoski (1984); $N = 99$
	10%-14% experienced depression of clinical severity at 3 days postpartum	Manly, McMahon, Bradley, &Davidson (1982); $N = 50$
	6.1% with major depression and 10.4% with minor depression at 8 weeks postpartum	Whiffen (1988); $N = 115$

antidepressant medications (over a period of months) before they found one that alleviated her symptoms.

I started to lose the ability to talk to anyone for more than a few minutes. When trying to communicate, I felt tightness in my chest and just wanted to cry. I continued to lose my ability to take care of the children and needed help for this task from my parents. All I could do was lie in bed and cry. The more I cried, the more anxious I got. I felt I hurt my family by not being able to function for them, and yet I must reinforce the fact that I was unable to take care of the baby, my older son, house, or husband. I was disappointed that I was missing my daughter's young baby days. One minute I would say, "Baby, you and I got cheated." The next minute, I would feel angry and feel like hitting her, and then I would run upstairs and cry.

Finally, in December, out of frustration I began sitting in dark closets to cry, running barefoot through the snow, sleeping in the bathtub, and pouring tea over my head. These tasks were done in order to release anxiety which had gone out of control and felt similar to a drug addict going straight.

As data in Table 1.2 indicate, the incidence of postpartum depression occurs in roughly 10%-40% of women (Thirkettle & Knight, 1985). The variation in the reported incidence of depression may be due in part to the lack of standardized assessment strategies for diagnosing depression and the differences in definitions of depression (Hopkins et al., 1984). For example, O'Hara et al. (1984) differentiated between the *syndrome* of postpartum depression and the *symptoms* of depression. O'Hara et al. felt that studies that relied on symptoms may have overestimated the rate of postpartum depression because normal physiological changes of pregnancy and puerperium may be reflected as depression symptoms (e.g., loss of sexual interest, fatigue, change in appetite). Conversely Affonso and Arizmendi (1986) argued that these symptoms were important indicators. For example, all new mothers can expect to feel fatigue, but mothers who were not at risk for depression coped more effectively with their fatigue and made a more successful postpartum adjustment. Affonso and Arizmendi further stated that clinicians often overlook depression because the symptoms of it are seen as "normal" concomitants of childbirth.

The Blues Versus Postpartum Depression

The relationship of the blues to depression also has been of interest to researchers. Two studies (Cox, Connor, & Kendell,

1982; Hapgood et al., 1988) found that the blues were significantly correlated with postnatal depression but that the relationship between these conditions was not always clear. In the first study, puerperal lability of mood was a better predictor of psychiatric symptoms up to 14 months later than were tears, sadness, or depression (Hapgood et al., 1988). In the Cox et al. (1982) study, 16% of the women in the sample were depressed within the first 10 days postpartum, a finding that contradicts the idea that depression starts later than the blues. Another study found that the blues were associated only with postpartum depression in the absence of stressful life events (Paykel, Emms, Fletcher, & Rassaby, 1980). The authors concluded that their findings suggest a small subgroup of women for whom hormonal factors are the cause.

Although there appears to be a relationship between the blues and postpartum depression, we do not know whether the blues *cause* later depression or whether they simply share common causal factors. Moreover we do not know whether the blues are an independent risk factor or an early stage of depression (O'Hara, 1987). The two conditions have considerable overlap between symptoms, including sadness, tearfulness, anxiety, and lability of mood. As a practical matter, O'Hara (1987) suggested that clinicians focus on the severity of symptoms rather than on trying to differentiate particularly between the blues and depression. Time that clinicians waste trying to distinguish between these two conditions precludes early intervention. It also can exacerbate a woman's symptoms by making her feel more isolated and alienated from people who could help.

Postpartum Psychosis

The first week postpartum was when the mania and psychosis started to show. I wasn't eating or sleeping well. I had a hard time completing a task, like feeding the baby. By 2 weeks postpartum, I was out of touch with the baby. It was extreme mania. Others would feed her. I lost control. . . . I had lots of energy in the middle of the night. All of a sudden I had to have all my announcements done, all my thank-you notes done. Everything was important to me. Dates from high school. I looked for connections with everything. I called friends I hadn't spoken to in years. . . . [After being taken to the emergency room]

TABLE 1.3 Postpartum Psychosis: Timing of Onset, Symptoms, and Incidence

Topic	Major findings	References
Onset	Typically within 2-4 weeks or as late as 8 weeks postpartum	Ifabumuyi & Akindele (1985); Snaith (1983)
Duration	Depends on diagnosis and treatment prescribed	Davidson & Robertson (1985)
Symptoms	Heightened or reduced motor activity; hallucinations; marked deviation in mood; severe depression, mania, or both; confusion; delirium	Leathe (1987); Stern & Kruckman (1983); Thirkettle & Knight (1985)
Incidence	1 to 2 per 1000 postpartum women	Mueller (1985); Stern & Kruckman (1983)

the doctor in the ER restrained me. I bit one of the supervisors, so he put me on Haldol to calm me down. He sent me to the psych hospital for 8 days. . . . I felt like I had no control. I was like a wild dog. All of a sudden I went from being a normal person having a baby, to a completely different person [Christine].

The most severe of the postpartum illnesses is postpartum psychosis. *Postpartum psychosis* is defined in terms of its severity and the vivid presentation of symptoms. The research on symptoms, incidence, and timing of onset is summarized in Table 1.3.

In two studies of women hospitalized for severe postpartum illness in Edinburgh, Scotland (Davidson & Robertson, 1985), and Kaduna, Nigeria (Ifabumuyi & Akindele, 1985), the three most common diagnoses were unipolar depression, bipolar depression, and schizophrenia. Transient organic psychosis was also a diagnosis for a small percentage of subjects in both studies.

As in the case of postpartum depression, it is debatable whether postpartum psychosis is distinct from nonpostpartum psychosis. O'Hara (1987), in his review of the literature, concluded that the evidence so far does not suggest a distinction between the two, except that postpartum psychosis occurs shortly after childbirth. Further, postpartum psychosis is no longer a separate diagnostic category in the *International Classification of Diseases* (ICD-9) or the *Diagnostic and Statistical Manual* (DSM).

In contrast Schoepf, Bryois, Jonquiere, and Scharfetter (1985) found that first-degree relatives of patients with nonpostpartum episodes of psychosis were much more likely to have psychotic episodes than were patients who only had postpartum psychosis. The authors indicated that their findings suggest postpartum psychosis *is distinct* from nonpostpartum psychosis. At the present time, however, postpartum psychosis is diagnosed and treated in the same ways as are episodes of nonpostpartum psychosis. Hospitalization and medications are generally required in these cases.

Even though this is a serious condition, the prognosis for most women suffering from postpartum psychosis is good. Two follow-up studies of women who had suffered from severe postpartum illness requiring hospitalization showed that the likelihood for recovery was good for all postpartum conditions except schizophrenia that develops in the puerperium (Davidson & Robertson, 1985; Mueller, 1985). Mueller (1985) discovered, however, that 65% of 57 women who were reexamined several years after their initial hospitalization had suffered at least one nonpostpartum relapse of their illness. Nevertheless postpartum psychosis appears to respond well to antipsychotic medications, and the majority of women recover (Snaith, 1983).

INFANTICIDE AND SUICIDE

Perhaps the most shocking reaction to postpartum illness is when a mother takes her own life or that of her baby. Scott (1987) characterized these responses as the "extreme tip of the iceberg" in terms of postpartum depression. Unfortunately we know very little about this from scientific inquiry. Most of what we know is based on anecdotal evidence and clinical reports. Nevertheless these anecdotal reports do shed some light on this frightening response.

For example, Angela Thompson became delusional after she stopped nursing her son at age 9 months. She drowned him in the bathtub after hearing the voice of God tell her that the child was the devil (Toufexis, 1988). In a Southern California case, Sheryl Massip drove over her 6-week-old son after being compelled to by voices in her head (Lachnit, 1990). In other cases of infanticide, however, the link between women killing their children and postpartum illness is less clear. For example, Lucrezia

Gentile drowned her 2-month-old son because she could not stand his incessant crying. Kathleen Householder hit her 2-week-old daughter with a rock because she was fussing. And Michele Remington shot her infant son before she tried to take her own life (Toufexis, 1988). In these cases it is less clear whether these infant deaths are because of fatal child abuse or are reactions to postpartum illness.

The results of one study indicate that the incidence of infanticide as a reaction to postpartum depression appears to be low (Davidson & Robertson, 1985). What may be more common are obsessional thoughts about harming the baby. We do not know how many women experience these types of thoughts, however, because incidence and prevalence studies have not been conducted. Five women of the 22 who shared their stories for this book, however, spontaneously described these thoughts and indicated that they occurred on many occasions. Interestingly only one of the women had symptoms of postpartum psychosis (and even this was never officially diagnosed). Yet all of the women were under severe stress from a colicky, crying baby (Barbara); traumatic birth experience (DeeDee); severe postpartum fatigue (Charlotte); the deaths of two people in her family shortly after she gave birth (Dawn); or a past history of child sexual abuse (Val). The stories of Barbara, Charlotte, and DeeDee are summarized below:

> Sometimes I'd walk by knives in the kitchen, and I'd think about killing her. I never told anyone about these thoughts, not even my husband until recently. I sometimes have these [same thoughts] happen before my period [Barbara].

> I began to think that my daughter was brain-damaged and would die at 5 weeks or 10 weeks. I also thought that because she was a girl, she would suffer as I had suffered and would be better off dead. I had thoughts of ending her life "humanely" by suffocating her. These thoughts terrified me. I became anxious about everything, unable to experience any joy or hope. I felt strangely detached from her and that she was a "bad," worthless baby, the total opposite of my older daughter, who had given me so much joy. I prayed for the world to end so that I wouldn't have to kill myself or my child [Charlotte].

> My postpartum depression was basically weird thoughts toward the baby, and he was a wonderful baby. The perfect baby. One time

I had him on the bathroom floor with me. All of a sudden, I had this thought to kick the baby. This was the first weird thought I had toward him. My pediatrician told me that this was very normal. "You had a traumatic delivery." . . . I would have weird thoughts when I was breast-feeding. I was constantly worried that the baby would hit his head on the table. I was also scared to walk through the doorway, that he would hit his head. These thoughts would become obsessive. I was afraid if I told anyone, they'd take the baby away. I finally told my mom. She said it was normal and not to worry. This lasted around 5 months. . . . If I was ironing, I'd be terrified that the baby would be burned. Even if he was upstairs asleep in his bed. Then I would start to analyze my thoughts. "Am I thinking he'd be burned because I wanted him to be burned?" I was also scared of knives. . . . I didn't want to do these things. I couldn't understand why I was thinking this way. . . . These thoughts happened every day, all the time. Slowly I had fewer thoughts. I'd think, "There's no way he can hit his head when I'm holding him." Around 1 year, I was scared of giving him a bath. I saw an Oprah [Oprah Winfrey show] about women who killed their babies. One woman drowned her baby in the bath at around 1 year. . . . The hardest thing was I couldn't find anyone who had this experience. I knew about it, but I couldn't seem to find anyone who had been through it [DeeDee].

Maternal suicide is another startling and tragic reaction to postpartum illness. It is often even more difficult to establish a link between postpartum illness and suicide because it might not occur until several months after a woman has a baby. A recent California case demonstrates this point. Victoria Karter, age 33, checked into the Four Seasons Hotel and jumped to her death 5 months after the birth of her daughter (Kalfus & Shaffer, 1990). Perhaps the most shocking aspect of this case is that Mrs. Karter committed suicide when outside observers would have described her as having a complete and happy life: stable marital relationship, good relationship with her family, and beautiful new baby. But Mrs. Karter's depression had been increasingly severe over the previous several months, and she had been in treatment for postpartum depression.

Suicide following postpartum depression is also relatively rare, according to the results of the only empirical study that has examined this issue (Davidson & Robertson, 1985). As with thoughts of harming the baby, however, we do not know the incidence or prevalence of suicidal ideation. Three of the mothers whom we spoke with indicated they had these types of thoughts:

I'm still dealing with the sexual abuse [her own past history]. I hadn't dealt with it before the birth. I told my husband [for the first time] in the hospital. I was hysterical. . . . I was afraid of being alone, so my husband stayed the night. If I could've opened the window, I would have jumped out [Val].

I had breast-feeding problems. He was colicky. I was afraid I wouldn't be able to comfort him. I didn't have thoughts of hurting him, but I thought of suicide. That's how depressed I was [Elizabeth].

The severe depression would come on and go away. One time I was sorting through all our medicines, sorting the ones that were very lethal into a pile. The severe episodes only lasted about half a minute, but the moderate depression stayed. I couldn't be left alone [Melissa].

Davidson and Robertson (1985) conducted perhaps the only empirical study of infanticide and suicide in puerperal women. They followed 82 patients who had been hospitalized for postpartum illness between 1946 and 1971. Of these 82 women with severe postpartum reactions, 52% were diagnosed with unipolar depression, 18% with bipolar depression, 16% with schizophrenia, and 11% with other mental illnesses. Of this group of women, all of whom had been affected severely by postpartum illness, 5% ultimately committed suicide, and the probable incidence of infanticide was 4% (some of the cases had not been confirmed). Of the patients who committed suicide, two had unipolar depression and two were schizophrenic. Only one of the suicides occurred during the postpartum illness, one took place after 3 years, and the other two took place after 12 years. One woman with unipolar depression was known to have committed infanticide, and another was strongly suspected to have done so. One of the schizophrenic women killed her two youngest children 18 months after the onset of her first symptoms after childbirth.

The results of this study indicate that infanticide and suicide are relatively rare, even among this most seriously affected subgroup of postpartum women. Despite the rarity of infanticide and suicide, we should remember that the possibility exists and should take appropriate steps. In the next section we recommend several types of actions that you can take.

SUGGESTIONS FOR NURSES

The following suggestions stem from several sources, including our background in crisis intervention, our experiences interviewing women on a variety of sensitive issues including postpartum depression, and suggestions from local clinicians who specialize in postpartum illness. Some of the suggestions apply mainly to nurses who have contact with mothers after they leave the hospital, because many of these symptoms may not appear for weeks or even months after delivery.

Recognition of Symptoms

As nurses, you are likely to be the only professionals with whom the majority of postpartum women have contact. Even if your contact is relatively brief, it may be the only link between mothers and sources of help. The symptoms of postpartum illness are often vague and may seem to be merely exaggerations of normal reactions to childbirth. Therefore you may need to read between the lines when talking with women and to take care not to discount all feelings as the blues. Some symptoms that you should pay particular attention to are when women say that they feel overwhelmed, that nothing will ever be the same, or that they feel hopeless or out of control. Also be alert to the possibility that a woman is suffering from depression if she is describing anxiety, nervousness, or insomnia (especially early-morning waking).

Mothers may be very reluctant to bring up these issues on their own. We have found it helpful to ask very specific questions to find out how women feel. Sometimes using a written list of questions will help gather the information you need, or using a questionnaire such as the *Edinburgh Postnatal Depression Scale*[2] will reveal depression. General questions such as, "How's everything going?" are likely to elicit responses like "Fine," with no further elaboration about their distress. Examples of more effective questions are, "Have you been feeling sad?" "Have you been crying lately?" "How much?" "Do you feel that you are a good mother?" "Are you enjoying the baby?" Sometimes even asking these types of questions can validate a woman's feelings and give her permission to tell you how she really feels.

Responding to Suicidal Threats

Take all suicide threats or reports of suicidal thoughts seriously. Although puerperal suicide is relatively rare, the possibility does exist. Suicide experts suggest asking any woman who indicates that she has had thoughts of suicide specific questions about how far her plans have progressed for committing suicide—for example, "What methods would you use?" Contact your local suicide-prevention hot line for information about how best to proceed and for referrals of people who can help. Ignoring someone's talk of suicide can be dangerous.

Responding to Concerns About Infant Harm

Descriptions of thoughts about harming the baby also must be handled with great care, even though it might make you upset when women tell you about them. The women whom we spoke with indicated that professionals often reacted with either great alarm or by assuring the mothers that the thoughts were "normal." The women who were troubled by these thoughts indicated that one of the worst reactions people had was to become alarmed and express great concern that they would kill their babies. This reaction did not stop the thoughts but actually fed into them and made them more intense.

It is equally unhelpful when professionals dismiss these thoughts as "normal," because the women themselves know that they are not. They may be fairly commonplace, but that does not mean they are normal. We suggest taking these thoughts seriously but not hitting the panic button. First, say in a neutral but concerned tone, "It must be very distressing to you to have such thoughts. Many other women have these thoughts, and they do not mean that you are a bad mother or will harm your baby. These thoughts usually mean that you are under some type of stress, and it may help to talk with someone about it." Then you can offer some names of people who can help. This type of approach validates her experience, while taking the problem seriously.

In more serious cases, you may need to take additional action. If the mother refuses help, or if you fear that the baby is in danger, you may be legally obligated to make a report to the Department of Social Services or the local child protective agency.

In the next chapter we describe the physiological causes of postpartum depression and psychosis.

NOTES

1. *Depressive symptoms* are not always synonymous with "the blues." Depressive symptoms is a term that reflects an entity distinct from the more serious syndrome of postpartum depression.

2. The entire *Edinburgh Postnatal Depression Scale* (EPDS) is found in the appendix of Cox, Holden, & Sagovsky (1987). The EPDS is a 10-item self-administered questionnaire that can be used to screen for postpartum depression (and to supplement your own clinical judgment). Instructions for scoring are included within the appendix of the Cox et al. article, and individuals are given permission to reproduce this scale. It is also available from Depression After Delivery (see the Appendix of this book for the address and telephone number). We highly recommend this easy-to-use questionnaire.

TWO

Physiological Factors

My counselor felt that it was all hormonal—about 80% biochemical. I do too now. I know fatigue played a big part. My counselor helped me see that. I nursed each [child], up to two times a night, so my sleep was constantly being interrupted. My husband gave our last baby a bottle at night. The depression was not as severe this time, and the only things I am doing differently are that my husband gave the baby a bottle, and I had someone to talk with [Debbie].

When seeking to understand postpartum depression, professionals and lay people alike often look toward physiological explanations. In many ways this is a sensible approach. The puerperium is a time of tremendous physiological change. A massive drop in progesterone and estrogen, and a corresponding increase in prolactin occur. Also ensuing are dramatic weight loss, a drop in blood volume, breast engorgement, and physical recovery from vaginal or cesarean birth. And these changes all take place within a few days of each other. Moreover, postpartum depression occurs when everyone expects a woman to be so happy. If no obvious environmental triggers to depression can be found, then clinicians assume that the explanation must be endogenous. The confidence that people place in physiological explanations is reflected in the following quotations:

Postpartum blues may be partially caused by a sudden drop in the level of endorphins, a substance released in the brain. (Bennett, 1990, p. 6)

The most common explanation for these postpartum disorders is dramatic hormonal changes in the body and brain before, during, and after childbirth. (Moore, 1990, p. 34)

Several theories currently address the actual cause of PPD; however, the root of the problem in almost all cases is hormonal. (Leathe, 1987, p. 74)

In this chapter we examine three possible physiological causes of depression: hormonal changes, physical pain, and fatigue. The first explanation—hormonal changes—is by far the most common.

HORMONES AND DEPRESSION: THE RAGING CONTROVERSY

Each [episode of] depression had very severe depression and anxiety initially. It was unmistakably chemical or hormonal. I could feel it hit. It was like someone injecting cold into my veins, and I could feel it up to my brain, a very strong physical sensation. The second time, I went home [from the hospital] with a prescription of Xanax. I had one episode and took it [the Xanax] for a week, and it took care of it. . . . I also had chills, fever, and diarrhea when the physical sensations hit. . . . There really was a physical component [Melissa].

Of all theories, the hormonal theory of postpartum depression has most captured the imagination of clinicians, researchers, and lay people alike. At present we know that women undergo substantial changes in hormone levels in the immediate postpartum period. The bone of contention, however, is whether these changes are related to depression. Past research has produced mixed results.

The most well studied hormones in relation to postpartum depression are estrogen and progesterone. Depression is hypothesized as being most likely to occur if estrogen and progesterone levels are low (O'Hara, 1987). (Sometimes the metabolites of estrogen—e.g., estriol and estradiol—are examined separately.) This explanation is popular because the large drop in the levels of these hormones is directly related to childbirth and the subsequent absence of the placenta (Dalton, 1971) and has been used to explain the blues, depression, and psychosis.

A more recent line of inquiry has focused on the hypotha-
lamic-pituitary-adrenal axis, particularly the role of cortisol
levels in postpartum mood disturbances. Cortisol has received
much less attention than have estrogen and progesterone, but
recent studies often have included all three in their analyses.
Increased levels of cortisol are thought to be related to postpartum depression because it has been noted that nonpuerperally
depressed patients have high levels of cortisol (Stern & Kruckman, 1983). The findings on the effects of estrogen, progesterone, and cortisol are described below.

The Synchronicity of Onset

> Two days after the baby was born, the depression started. I was
> discharged that day. On the third day, I was fine. It hit all of a
> sudden. It wasn't severe until the fifth day. I knew enough this
> time to make myself eat, make myself sleep. But I still couldn't
> control the crying. I knew immediately what was wrong. I had
> medications left from last time. I immediately called my psychia-
> trist and started the medication [Julie].

In a study of 81 women during the first 3 weeks after childbirth, Kendell, McGuire, Connor, and Cox (1981) found a day-5
peak for self-reported ratings of depression, tears, and lability.
This peak occurred regardless of when women left the hospital,
for primiparous and multiparous women, for breast- and bot-
tle-feeders, and for women who had caesarean or vaginal deliveries (Kendell, MacKenzie, West, McGuire, & Cox, 1984).
Because the peak was so consistent across women in their
sample, regardless of life circumstances, the authors felt that it
suggests a hormonal explanation. Less postpartum mood disturbance was found among women who left the hospital within
48 hours after delivery, however, suggesting at least some mediating effect of the environment.
    In a study of 43 Jamaican women, Davidson (1972) found that
60.4% of these women experienced some emotional upset during the first 11 days postpartum, most of which occurred on
days 1-3. In a prospective study of 105 women (Cox et al., 1982),
the authors noted that psychiatric symptoms are at their highest
in the 10 days after delivery. This is when the fall in estrogen

and progesterone are maximal. The authors felt that this and the failure to find any connection with social factors, marital relationship, or obstetric complications give indirect support for the endocrine hypothesis.

The results of the above-cited studies suggest that the blues and depression are likely to occur when corresponding changes occur in levels of hormones in the puerperium. Because the blues develop for so many women and in a variety of life circumstances, some have argued that this suggests a hormonal explanation. Others, however, have argued against a hormonal explanation and point out that the blues are not unique to the puerperium.

In one recent study Levy (1987) compared emotional reactions of puerperal women ($N = 37$), women who had had major surgery ($N = 28$), and women who had had minor surgery ($N = 22$). Her results revealed a similar pattern of distress for the puerperal women and for women who had had major surgery. In fact more dysphoria occurred after major surgery than after childbirth. Further, crying and depression peaked in the same way in the postoperative women as it did in the puerperal women, with many postoperative patients commenting that the blues occurred suddenly and unexpectedly around the fourth postoperative day.

In summary, in spite of some evidence for the day-5 peak, a number of factors argue against a wholly hormonal explanation for the blues (Chalmers & Chalmers, 1986). For example, not every mother experiences these emotions, which we would expect because all mothers experience hormonal readjustments (Manly, McMahon, Bradley, & Davidson, 1982). Further, in some cultures the majority of women do not experience the blues, a phenomenon suggesting a strong mediating effect of the environment (Stern & Kruckman, 1983). In addition, fathers and women who adopt children often experience the blues and depression but do not experience hormonal adjustments.

Hormone Levels in Depressed and Nondepressed Women

Another line of inquiry has focused on comparing hormone levels between depressed and nondepressed women. In one study (Feksi, Harris, Walker, Riad-Fahmy, & Newcomb, 1984) the authors compared the hormone levels found in the saliva of five women with severe blues with those of women who were symptom free for 5 days postpartum. The saliva samples were assayed by people blind to the status of the women (depressed versus nondepressed). On the day that the women showed symptoms, women in the "severe blues" group had significantly higher levels of estradiol and progesterone than did the symptom-free women. The groups did not differ in their levels of cortisol, however. The authors made a case for using saliva samples for assessing hormone levels; most researchers, however, continue to assess these levels by using blood samples.

In a study of nomifensine treatment (a tetrahydro-isoquinoline antidepressant), the authors found no difference in the pretreatment levels of estradiol and progesterone in eight depressed women and eight nondepressed controls (Butler & Leonard, 1986). The levels of these hormones were unaffected by the treatment even though the nomifensine alleviated symptoms. The authors did notice that depression seemed to be related to serotonin levels (specifically the H-serotonin uptake rates) rather than specific hormones per se that underlie postpartum depression.

Dalton has been one of the most active and outspoken proponents of the view that the sudden drop in progesterone is responsible for postpartum mood disturbance. She gave progesterone prophylactically to 100 women who had previous episodes of postpartum depression (Dalton, 1985). A recurrence of postnatal depression occurred in nine women (10%), compared with a recurrence rate of 68% in 221 women who had experienced postnatal depression previously and had received no progesterone. It should be noted that this was not a double-blind design. We have no way of determining whether the alleviation of symptoms was the result of progesterone therapy or a placebo effect. In fact another group of researchers (VanderMeer, Loendersloot, & VanLoenen, 1984) did conduct a double-blind placebo controlled trial comparing the effect of progesterone suppositories with a placebo on ten women suffering from postpartum depression. No significant difference was found between the effect of the progesterone and the effect of the placebo. Indeed, when comparing subjective effects, three of the women preferred the placebo.

Two researchers (Dalton, 1971; Pitt, 1968) noted a relationship between menstrual problems (dysmenorrhea and premenstrual

[handwritten: PMS + menopause = PPD]

syndrome) and postpartum depression, again suggesting a hormonal link. They felt that their results suggest postpartum depression is caused by women's bodies not making adequate adjustments to massive hormonal changes occurring after giving birth. Conversely, Davidson (1972) and O'Hara, Rehm, and Campbell (1982) failed to find any connection between menstrual difficulties and mild or severe postpartum depression.

In perhaps the most carefully controlled and comprehensive study to date, O'Hara, Schlechte, Lewis, and Varner (1991) drew blood and urine samples from approximately 173 women (number of participants varied slightly from assessment to assessment) at 34, 36, and 38 weeks gestation and at days 1, 2, 3, 4, 6, and 8 postpartum. The authors studied levels of estradiol, free estriol, progesterone, prolactin, total cortisol, and urinary free cortisol. The depressed subjects in their sample ($N = 18$) showed significantly lower levels of estradiol at 36 weeks gestation and at Day 2 postpartum but no other significant differences. Specifically, no significant differences were found in levels of free estriol, total estriol, progesterone, prolactin, total plasma cortisol, or urinary free cortisol between depressed and nondepressed subjects at any of the other assessment periods. Further, no significant differences were found between depressed and nondepressed subjects for ratios of prolactin to estradiol or progesterone for any of the assessments. The authors concluded that there was little evidence of a hormonal influence in postpartum depression.

The Role of Prolactin

> The panic attacks were isolated until I quit nursing. Two days after discontinuing the nursing, the panic attacks came without warning and furiously. That's why I also think [my depression] is basically hormonal [Barbara].

In addition to studying the effects of sex hormones and cortisol, some researchers have studied the effects of prolactin. According to this view, depression is likely to occur when prolactin levels are too high. Prolactin levels increase with the onset of lactation (Susman & Katz, 1988). Researchers have noted a connection between high levels of prolactin and depression, anxiety, and hostility in the puerperium.

Kellner, Buckman, M. Fava, G. Fava, and Mastrogiacomo (1984) reviewed the research on prolactin to date, but they only included studies that used the *Symptom Questionnaire*. All four studies (*N* = approximately 10) found that higher prolactin levels were associated with higher hostility ratings (as indicated by scores on the *Symptom Questionnaire*). Depression and anxiety levels also were associated with high levels of prolactin. Two studies compared hyperprolactinemic amenorrheic women with amenorrheic women who had normal prolactin levels, or hyperprolactinemic women with normal controls. Hyperprolactinemic postpartum women were more hostile than either nonpostpartum hyperprolactinemic women or normal controls. When bromocriptine, a prolactin-lowering drug, was administered to hyperprolactinemic women in a double-blind study, a decrease in hostility, depression, and anxiety occurred that corresponded with the decrease in prolactin. No such change occurred with the placebo. The authors of the review postulated that hostility associated with high prolactin levels may be a vestige of an evolutionary advantage for women protecting their young. This idea is highly speculative, however, and runs counter to the common notion that prolactin increases maternicity (Sears, 1991). Finally, an in-depth study of four women (Susman & Katz, 1988) also noted a connection between weaning and postpartum mood disturbance. The authors of this study pointed out, however, that three of these four women also had family histories of affective disorders.

Conclusions

Researchers to date have not established that puerperal hormonal changes cause the blues, depression, or psychosis (Stern & Kruckman, 1983). In fact even consistent correlational evidence is missing, with several studies finding that hormone levels are correlated with depression, and other studies finding no such relation (O'Hara, 1987). Many of the existing studies that have found differences used small samples of women, and some of the studies had serious methodological difficulties, including lack of control groups and lack of a double-blind design.

O'Hara et al. (1991) offered several explanations for the inconsistencies in findings regarding the effects of hormones. Past studies have been inconsistent in their use of assessment techniques and definitions of postpartum illness. It also may be possible that only the most severely affected women show hormone imbalances. Some studies have used samples of severely depressed women, while others have included both mildly and severely depressed women in their samples, perhaps obscuring results.

Future research should move beyond examining the effects of individual hormones and should examine these effects within the context of the entire endocrine or limbic systems. Further, depression should be examined in relation to key neurotransmitters such as serotonin and norepinephrine. Clearly more comprehensive and carefully controlled studies must be conducted before we can declare that hormones are a major cause of postpartum depression. In conclusion we should proceed with caution about our use of hormone replacement therapy and should be aware that current evidence does not support prophylactic use of hormones for preventing or treating postpartum depression.

POSTPARTUM PAIN AND DEPRESSION

I was surprised at how sore I was. Friends seem to recover quickly. I wasn't expecting it to hurt so much [DeeDee].

The link between pain after childbirth and postpartum depression has not been extensively examined. Davidson (1972) noted that postpartum pain was significantly related to incidence of the blues for women in his sample, and Snaith (1983) described it as a possible cause of depression. Researchers also have explored the relation between chronic pain and depression in general.

After childbirth women may experience pain from a variety of sources: incisions following cesarean birth, gas pains, swollen breasts, episiotomies and/or perineal lacerations, uterine contractions, or muscle aches and pains. This pain is often chronic albeit temporary. Even though it is temporary, it can be overwhelming and frightening and can contribute to postpartum depression. Julie had pain from an unexpected postpartum complication. This was her first episode of postpartum depression and her second birth:

I've had [depression] with two of my three children. With the first depression, I had a paravaginal hematoma the size of a softball. It developed 12 hours after birth. After that, it abscessed. I was in the hospital 7-8 days because they couldn't get my fever down. . . . It was hard to be in the hospital. I just had a baby, but you'd never know it. I never saw him. I don't even remember the first 6 months of his life. I was pregnant all that time and had nothing to show for it. . . . All I remember is excruciating pain and a long time in the hospital and not being able to bond with my baby, not feeling like a mother. . . . With the first depression, I was embarrassed, I didn't want to tell others. It was mental illness, and people were afraid of it. . . . I had uncontrollable crying for no reason, problems with my appetite. I'd worry about little things, I didn't want to take care of the baby or anybody. I was overwhelmed. . . . My psychiatrist thought that having to be rehospitalized made the depression worse and last longer. He felt I was traumatized by the rehospitalization.

Several factors can influence whether a stimulus is perceived as painful, including fatigue and loss of sleep, decreased nutritional intake, and anxiety and fear. Anxiety and fear send messages to the cerebral cortex, which amplifies impulses sent to the thalamus, thereby increasing the perception of pain. When pain is perceived as intense, it increases anxiety and fear. Anxiety and fear increase the perception of pain, setting off a vicious cycle of pain and fear (Affonso & Walpole, 1979).

The perception of pain can be influenced also by social and cultural variables. For example, members of different ethnic groups have different responses to pain. In research comparing responses after surgery, Jewish and Italian patients were more open about expressing the amount of pain that they were in, while those of Anglo-Saxon or Irish background tended to be more stoic, detached, and matter-of-fact (Zborowski, 1969). Therefore women's social or cultural backgrounds can influence the meaning they attach to pain, which can affect how much pain they feel (Zimbardo, 1985). Other evidence for the psychosocial influences on the perception of pain is the placebo effect. Believing that you are getting something that will relieve your pain is often enough to release the pain-killing endorphins in the brain, which make the stimulus less painful (Lahey, 1992).

In terms of psychological impact, pain can lead to a sense of helplessness (Affonso & Walpole, 1979) and depression (Gildenberg, 1984). *Learned helplessness* has been conceptualized as the mechanism through which pain causes depression in individuals. The concept of learned helplessness was first developed from a series of animal studies in which animals received shocks and were prevented from escaping. When animals could escape in later phases of the experiment, the dogs that had been previously shocked were slower to learn the response that stopped the shock or slower to try to escape than were animals who had had no prior shock (Seligman & Maier, 1967).

Learned helplessness applied to humans refers to a lack of effort to avoid negative events, which often is caused by previous exposure to unavoidable negative events (Lahey, 1992). When humans are faced with a situation that seems inescapable, they become depressed, which leads them not to try to escape or change the noxious circumstances (Seligman, 1972). When people feel trapped or overwhelmed by pain, their response may be to become depressed. This effect has been demonstrated in studies of people with chronic pain (e.g., Atkinson, Ingram, Kremer, & Saccuzzo, 1986; Kroetsch, & Shamoian, 1983).

Pain of unknown origin can be frightening, and women may fear that they will "always" feel this way. These feelings are especially difficult when women suddenly are forced to take care of a demanding newborn when they want someone else to take care of them. If women accept this pain as "the way it is," they may not be motivated to try to alleviate it. Rathus (1991) pointed out that education is an important component in the management of chronic pain. When patients know the origin of their pain and have an idea of how long it will last and how much pain will be involved, they cope with the pain more effectively than do patients who feel overwhelmed and trapped by it. In addition, teaching women simple procedures they can do to alleviate their own pain can help them feel more in control of it (Affonso & Walpole, 1979). In summary it is important for women to learn as much as they can about their pain and ways for them to control it in order to minimize the risk of depression.

THE ROLE OF FATIGUE IN DEPRESSION AND PSYCHOSIS

Winter was a bad time—Christmas through March. Both of the kids got sick and were up almost every night. I was incapacitated. I started screaming, and I couldn't stop. . . . I attribute the depression more to lack of sleep. When the kids got sick, I got very little sleep and the depression would be worse. This is associated with winter, they are more likely to get sick then. My husband does all the night time stuff now. He has been a godsend. When I started getting sleep, it started getting better. . . . With the first baby, I was in bed, unable to sleep, having panic attack after panic attack. I was sure I'd never sleep again. I've always needed a lot of sleep. Even 7 hours is a deprivation. My first baby needed almost none. That made it worse. . . . One night, I almost threw him out the window. People try to minimize that and say, "At least you didn't," but I don't know. [Melissa].

Another physiological factor related to postpartum depression is *fatigue*. Fatigue is ubiquitous to new mothers, and interrupted sleep is a fact of life for the first few months after a baby is born. Gardner and Campbell (1991) recommended regular assessment of fatigue for all new mothers and noted that this assessment is particularly needed in the postpartum period.

Perhaps because fatigue is commonplace, it has not been adequately studied in relation to postpartum illness (Pitt, 1973). Lack of research exists despite observations that sleep disturbances and fatigue, both symptoms of postpartum depression, interfere with a mother's abilities to cope with her responsibilities (Affonso, 1979). However, these symptoms may be contributing causal factors of postpartum depression as well as symptoms. In a study of 68 postpartum women, the highest levels of fatigue were found among the younger mothers and those with less household help, two or three other children, child care problems, and lower levels of education (Gardner, 1991). As we describe in Chapter 4, many of the factors related to fatigue in Gardner's study also are related directly to postpartum illness. The lack of interest in fatigue as a contributing factor to postpartum illness is somewhat surprising because sleep deprivation has been studied in relation to both depression and delusional thinking in nonpostpartum women and men. We have included it in this chapter because of its prominence in anecdotal and clinical accounts of postpartum illness and because of its influence on depression in general.

Fatigue and Depression

One possible reason why fatigue has not been adequately studied is because some have argued it is not an accurate indicator of postpartum depression. For example, O'Hara et al. (1984) concluded that traditional measures of depression that include fatigue as a symptom (e.g., the *Beck Depression Inventory*) probably overestimate the percentage of women with postpartum depression because fatigue is a normal concomitant of childbirth. Conversely Affonso and Arizmendi (1986) noted that although fatigue is normal among postpartum women, women making a successful postpartum adjustment are more able to cope with their fatigue than are women having adjustment problems.

When describing the relationship between fatigue and depression, we often are left a with chicken-and-egg type of question, not knowing which came first. Fatigue can be both a symptom of depression and a cause. Atkinson (1985) found that for women in general, fatigue is "inseparably linked to depression" (p. 284). Fatigue may be the primary symptom of depression and can manifest itself as loss of interest in the world and loss of energy.

One obvious source of fatigue is sleep deprivation. People deprived of sleep are often more depressed, less energetic, and less friendly than they were prior to being deprived of sleep (Roediger, Rushton, Capaldi, & Paris, 1986). We often assume that fatigue in new mothers is caused by being awakened by an infant during the night. Yet depression and anxiety also can cause sleep deprivation. Atkinson (1985) observed that depression can cause restless sleep and that early morning waking is an important symptom of depression. Affonso (1979) noted this as a symptom of postpartum depression as well, and it is surprisingly often overlooked as a factor precipitating depression.

I didn't know how things like sleep deprivation would affect me. I was up three times a night, changing her three times a night. It wasn't fair. Suddenly, I was doing menial tasks for this little being I didn't like. . . . I told [my midwife] when I saw her that I had been having insomnia. She told me it was "normal" and that I would "sleep when I was tired enough." She never picked up on my depression. I didn't know who to talk to. They give you a handout on postpartum depression, but it doesn't really prepare you. It's like graduating from college without knowing how to read. I saw [my midwife] again at 6 months [postpartum] for a diaphragm fitting. That was really an excuse. I just wanted to make a connection again. I told her how bad I had been feeling over the past 6 months. She was really shocked [Karen].

As is true of the psychological impact of pain, the psychological impact of fatigue is best understood in terms of learned helplessness. If a woman feels overwhelmed and out of control, she may withdraw to protect herself, either through fatigue or depression. When women take control of their lives, they begin to feel both less tired and less depressed (Atkinson, 1985). Taking control may mean something as simple as setting limits on demands that others place on them, asking for help, and realizing that they have a right to their feelings.

Although sleep deprivation is the most obvious source of fatigue, another line of research examined the role of thyroid function in postpartum depression (Harris et al., 1989). This study included 147 subjects, 22 of whom were diagnosed with major depression. Thyroid function was assessed by measuring levels of free thyroxine (fT4), tri-iodothyronine (fT3), and thyrotrophin (TSH). At 6-8 weeks postpartum, a higher incidence of depression was found in women with thyroid dysfunction (but the relation was only significant on one of three measures of postpartum depression). Three of the eight mothers who were diagnosed with postpartum thyroid dysfunction had major depression and showed depression on all three scales. The authors concluded that postpartum thyroid dysfunction often goes undetected because the women attribute symptoms (if indeed they manifest any) to postpartum fatigue. This conclusion offers another justification for including fatigue as an important symptom of postpartum depression, contrary to the suggestion of O'Hara et al. (1984). The authors also suggested routine postpartum screening for thyroid dysfunction. An earlier study (Hayslip et al., 1988) had similar findings. The authors of this study followed 51 women for 6 months postpartum and noted substantial psychiatric morbidity in women who developed postpartum hypothyroidism. The symptoms they noted in particular included impaired concentration and memory and a subjective difficulty in performing work.

In summary, fatigue can either cause or be symptomatic of postpartum depression. These studies indicate that fatigue can be caused by lack of sleep due to the infant or by anxiety associated with depression. Fatigue also can be caused by anemia or thyroid dysfunction. Although fatigue is a "normal" part of being a new mother, practitioners should keep in mind that it may be a possible symptom of depression.

Fatigue and Psychosis

Fatigue and sleep deprivation have been related to delusional thinking and other psychotic symptoms in men and women. Is it any surprise that sleep deprivation could have this same effect on women who have recently given birth? Published accounts of postpartum psychosis (e.g., Dix, 1985; Skinner, 1991) and accounts given by women interviewed for this book often indicate that women had had very little sleep prior to the onset of postpartum psychosis. Often the symptoms these women experience are attributed to "hormones." But it is equally plausible that the psychosis was a result of biochemical changes resulting from lack of sleep. Charlotte describes her experience.:

> My second postpartum experience was a nightmare. I never had enough milk, no matter how much I ate, drank, or rested. My baby lost weight. I was exhausted. . . . I decided to wean my baby at 2 months because I was so exhausted and depressed. . . . [At 2 ½ months postpartum] my brain started to malfunction. I became extremely forgetful. I made odd mistakes unrelated to the normal stress of child care demands. I couldn't remember the names of common household objects. I used words inappropriately. Proper nouns were lost at random. At one point I could not recall my children's names. I made driving mistakes, cooking mistakes, child care mistakes. I was terrified that I was going to get hopelessly lost, burn my house down, or cause a fatal auto accident. It was as if my mind would "go to sleep" for a few seconds while I was engaged in some activity. . . .
> I thought about suicide, institutionalization, and separation from my family constantly. . . . That postpartum psychosis exists was such a revelation to me because in April I had experienced a week of near-total insomnia. During these truly sleepless nights, I had no control over my thoughts, as if my brain had been put in a food processor. The first half of a thought would be rational and the second half would be totally unrelated, nonsensical.

In a classic case study of sleep deprivation, a New York disc jockey named Peter Tripp showed many of the symptoms of postpartum psychosis. In January 1959, Tripp endeavored to stay awake for 200 hours in a glass booth in Times Square as a fund-raiser for the March of Dimes. Below are excerpts from the government report on what happened to him:

Almost from the first, the desire to sleep was so strong that Tripp was fighting to keep himself awake. After little more than 2 days and 2 nights, he began to have visual illusions; for example, he reported finding cobwebs in his shoes. By about 100 hours the simple daily tests that required only minimal mental agility and attention were a torture for him. He was having trouble remembering things, and his visual illusions were perturbing: he saw the tweed suit of one of the scientists as a suit of fuzzy worms. . . . The daily tests were almost unendurable for Tripp and those who were studying him. "He looked like a blind animal trying to feel his way through a maze." A simple algebraic formula that he had earlier solved with ease now required such superhuman effort that Tripp broke down, frightened at his inability to solve the problem, fighting to perform. Scientists saw the spectacle of a suave New York radio entertainer trying vainly to find his way through the alphabet.

By 170 hours the agony had become almost unbearable to watch. At times Tripp was no longer sure he was himself, and frequently tried to gain proof of his identity. Although he behaved as if he were awake, his brain wave patterns resembled those of sleep. In his psychotic delusions he was convinced that the doctors were in a conspiracy against him to send him to jail. . . . At the end of the 200 sleepless hours, nightmare hallucination and reality had merged, and he felt he was the victim of a sadistic conspiracy among the doctors. (Luce, 1966, pp. 19-20)

Tripp recovered fairly quickly after he received about 13 hours of sleep, but he complained of depression for about 3 months after. A number of his experiences were similar to those of women suffering from postpartum psychosis, including delusions, hallucinations, and paranoia. It is interesting too that this case study was on a man who would not be subject to the same hormonal influences common in postpartum or menstruating women, yet he manifested symptoms similar to postpartum psychosis. Another case study described by Roediger et al. (1986) indicated that a male high school student stayed awake for 264 hours without the ill effects that were apparent in the case of Peter Tripp (although he did experience fatigue, sleepiness, and irritability). The discrepancy between the experiences of these two men indicates, among other things, that not everyone who is sleep deprived shows symptoms of psychosis. This indication could explain why only a small percentage of postpartum women become psychotic. Indeed some people may be more vulnerable to the effects of sleep deprivation in the same way that different people require different amounts of sleep per night.

Fortunately the effects of sleep deprivation are short-lived; most people recover relatively quickly after a night or two of solid sleep (Lahey, 1992; Roediger et al., 1986), but depression might linger. For others the effects are longer lasting. Judy, a labor and delivery nurse, describes how sleeplessness preceded her bout with postpartum psychosis. She initially was diagnosed as schizophrenic, and this was later changed to bipolar depression. She was hospitalized for 28 days.

> In the months after her birth I often was easily overwhelmed. Fatigue did not vanish. Fears of losing her, my boys, and/or [my husband] grasped me frequently. . . . Exhaustion came, but I did not submit. After [my daughter] was asleep, thoughts bombarded me for hours only to awake alert at 4 or 5 a.m. . . . The week after the [childbirth education] seminar, sleeplessness continued. A whimper or sneeze from one of my children would jar me into a state of alertness. Racing thoughts about the deficits of the maternity care system in the U.S. or my childhood bombarded my mind. I'd enter their room . . . hoping one of the three would be awake. Usually they weren't, so I spent hours formulating and recording plans and ideas.
>
> As the week progressed, I became less functional. We delayed leaving for a camping trip Thursday night, since I was unable to accomplish packing. [My husband] received phone calls from relatives telling him of the strange content of the lengthy long-distance calls I'd placed. He forbid me to use the phone. I continued, though, because I sensed a great urgency about my thoughts.

Sleep deprivation alone does not explain the mania that often precedes the psychosis and that contributes to the sleep deprivation. It is likely due to a combination of biological and psychological stressors. Another possibility is that undetected postpartum depression, or the anxiety that often accompanies depression, is creating an inability to stay asleep.

Sleep deprivation is often overlooked as a possible cause of postpartum psychosis. Case studies of postpartum psychosis and the effects of sleep deprivation in general suggest that developing a more complete understanding of the role of sleep deprivation in postpartum psychosis would be a fruitful topic for future research. Indeed, future research might reveal a connection between lower levels of serotonin and postpartum psychosis, because serotonin also is related to sleep. But for now the role of sleep deprivation in postpartum psychosis remains an open question.

SUGGESTIONS FOR NURSES

A Note on Antidepressant Medications

Because so many clinicians favor a biological explanation for postpartum depression, antidepressant medications have become a popular course of treatment. It is not treatment without controversy, however, and you might wish to help mothers sort through the risks and benefits of this treatment option. Some additional factors to keep in mind are the severity of the symptoms, impairment of the woman's functioning, and the availability of other treatment options.

Some antidepressants, such as bromocriptine (also a lactation suppressant) and tricyclic antidepressants, work by normalizing hormone and neurotransmitter levels in depressed women (especially levels of serotonin and norepinephrine). Perhaps the most common medications used for postpartum depression are tricyclics. Examples of these include amitriptyline (Elavil), imipramine (Tofranil), desipramine (Norpramin), and nortriptyline (Pamelor). These medications do have some side effects, such as dry mouth, constipation, urinary hesitancy, blurred vision, and confusion (McGrath et al., 1990). In addition, these medications do pass into breast milk, although in lower concentrations than in the mother's bloodstream. The long-term effects of these medications on infants has not been studied, so it may not be wise for mothers on these medications to continue to nurse, and this warning is repeatedly mentioned in the *Physicians' Desk Reference*. Other treatments include Prozac (another type of antidepressant), lithium (for the treatment of bipolar depression), and antipsychotic medications, although these are less common.

Minor tranquilizers, such as Ativan, Serax, Xanax, and Klonopin, can be useful for alleviating some of the anxiety that often accompanies postpartum illness. These are helpful until the antidepressant medication takes effect. They pass through breast milk, however, and do accumulate in the bloodstream of infants.

Therefore breast-feeding is contraindicated for women taking these medications.

Although tranquilizers and antidepressant medication can be helpful, even lifesaving, care should be given when deciding whether to use them. Some women feel stigmatized while on medication, a response that contributes to their image of being "sick" (Dix, 1985). Further, the American Psychological Association's Task Force on Women and Depression concluded that use of antidepressants may encourage "dependency, passivity, and a victim psychology in women, which could reinforce depression over time" (McGrath et al., 1990, p. xiii). The authors of this report pointed out that depression is misdiagnosed at least 30%-50% of the time, with nonpsychiatrists prescribing antianxiety drugs instead of antidepressants. Moreover, antidepressants given to women are often improperly monitored, a situation that makes prescription drug misuse a real danger for women. In addition, research has failed to address the interaction between antidepressants and hormonal changes during the menstrual cycle or in the immediate postpartum period.

These side effects would seem relatively minor if medications were the only effective treatment option. Recent research, however, reveals that they are only one possible option. In cases of less severe depression, antidepressants and structural or cognitive therapy have shown about the same success rates (McGrath et al., 1990). Panic disorders also respond equally well to both cognitive/behavioral therapy and minor tranquilizers (Adler, 1991a). This is not to rule out the use of antidepressants, for indeed they can alleviate a great deal of suffering. It is to caution that, when antidepressants are used, they should be monitored carefully and used in conjunction with other treatments. Holden, Sagovsky, and Cox (1989) found that the effects of antidepressants were enhanced when combined with therapeutic listening and social support.

Pain Management and Depression

Nurses are in a strategic position to help women manage pain. Many nurses already do this routinely, because pain in the postpartum period can be considerable. Pain management is an integral part of nursing, and obstetrical nursing texts contain many suggestions for helping women with postpartum pain. We have limited our brief discussion to pain management as a way to prevent or overcome postpartum depression.

As we indicated earlier, the key to pain management is to help women gain control over their pain. This can be accomplished in two ways: first, by educating women about the sources of their pain and how long it might last; and second, by teaching women about some of the "home remedies" they might try to help with their discomfort, such as sitz baths, heat lamps, ice packs for breasts and the perineum, medications for hemorrhoidal discomfort, walking, relaxation techniques such as those used for labor pains, and the use of analgesics. These simple techniques can help mothers feel more in control and may help them avoid depression.

Helping Women Overcome Fatigue

An article by Gardner and Campbell (1991) contains a one-page questionnaire that nurses can use to assess women's levels of postpartum fatigue. This questionnaire, or simply asking women questions about the amount of help they have and how tired they feel, will help you determine whether fatigue is contributing to a woman's depression. Helping women overcome fatigue may be more difficult.

If a woman is very fatigued or already is suffering from depression, you might need to problem-solve with her about how she can get more rest. This might include having her ask for help from her husband, family members, and friends or hiring someone to help with child care or household chores. By discussing this with her, you might be giving her "permission" to ask others for help, whereas she might not have felt entitled to before. Some inexpensive options for help outside the family include hiring a teenager after school to help with chores and meal preparation and arranging to "share" child care or meal preparation with another family that lives nearby. Other options will depend on the resources available to her. By involving family, friends, or neighbors in the solution, you also are increasing the woman's connections with others, thereby decreasing the isolation she might feel.

For some women fatigue might be due to an inability to sleep because of depression or anxiety. Any signs of insomnia or early-morning waking should be considered as possible symptoms of depression. In this case you should make a referral to a mental-health specialist (preferably one knowledgeable about postpartum depression). Several women whom we spoke with found minor tranquilizers (such as Xanax) to be helpful for letting them get some rest when they were experiencing anxiety. Although this is helpful, it is not a long-term solution. Other options include increasing exercise or modifying their diets (see Atkinson, 1985 for suggestions). Sleeping pills and tranquilizers should be used sparingly, because they inhibit REM sleep; and lack of REM sleep may contribute even further to fatigue (Atkinson, 1985). Other suggestions for reducing anxiety are found in Chapters 5 and 7.

The Role of Diet

In general, women suffering from postpartum depression should be given a complete physical, including a CBC to screen for anemia, and a thyroid test (T4 and TSH). In addition, a promising new line of research has noted a relationship between a high carbohydrate diet, depression, and levels of serotonin. Serotonin is the neurotransmitter thought to be affected by circulating sex hormones (see Butler & Leonard, 1986) and is affected by antidepressant medication. A high carbohydrate diet has been found to relieve both the symptoms of depression (Wurtman & Wurtman, 1989) and PMS (Liebman, 1990) in controlled clinical trails. This research suggests that counseling women to modify their diets to include a high percentage of complex carbohydrates may help alleviate some of their symptoms. An excellent program that you might recommend is the Weight Watchers Plan for Nursing Mothers. It is balanced nutritionally and is high in carbohydrates. (The regular Weight Watchers program also is high in carbohydrates and is significantly less expensive than most of its competitors.) A dietary approach has the advantage of not causing side effects or stigmatization that other treatments might. It is also something that the woman can do for herself and can increase her sense of control.

In the next chapter we describe the connection between negative birth experiences and postpartum depression.

THREE

Negative Birth Experiences

I'm certain that my birth experience triggered my depression. I was a healthy, emotionally strong person. Suddenly, I lost my sense of control during childbirth. Since then it's been like an avalanche. Things that are normally fun don't interest me now. I just can't seem to put the trauma of that night to rest—I replay it frequently. I desperately want to piece together everything that I missed so that I can be satisfied and move on [Sally].

Why is one woman deeply troubled by her birthing experience, while another is not? Some claim that women have "unrealistic expectations" because of their "natural childbirth" classes (Eisenberg, Murkoff, & Hathaway, 1989; Stewart, 1985). Others tell women to stop dwelling on negative aspects of their birth experiences and to remind themselves that the goal of labor and delivery is a healthy baby (Chalmers & Chalmers, 1986; Dix, 1985).

Although women may report feeling that they "failed" during labor (Erb, Hill, & Houston, 1983) or that their birth was not as they expected (Knight & Thirkettle, 1987), these feelings do not fully explain negative reactions to birth. Some women describe their labors and deliveries in even stronger terms, likening their birth experiences to sexual assaults or describing themselves as being "mutilated" or "violated" (Goer, 1991; Wessel, 1983). This is hardly language that people expect when women describe a supposedly happy event.

Moreover, even in this era of "family-centered" birthing, many women feel overwhelmed by the hospital environment. This notion often surprises professionals, who see that hospital births have become more humane over the past 10-15 years. These professionals assume that negative birth experiences are a thing of the past. Yet most experiences reported throughout this chapter have taken place within the past few years (1989-1991). Further, some of the changes that hospitals have made have been merely cosmetic, as Barbara describes:

> In [town name], they have birthing rooms they make a big deal about. You can have your baby in the room and there's nice wallpaper on the wall. *Big deal!* . . . I felt like a piece of meat in a meat market. I'm really angered. I don't think women should have to go through this.

By and large, researchers have approached the issue of women's reactions to birth rather naively. For example, most surgeons are aware that depression often occurs after major surgery, but this same assumption is not made about cesarean section (Levy, 1987; Oakley, 1983). Women are supposed to feel happy after this procedure because their babies are safe—and the vast majority of women are (see Erb et al., 1983). But there is denial that women might also have negative reactions. When women do voice their concerns, other people often react as if, by complaining, the women would have preferred the death or injury that could have followed if there had been no medical intervention (Oakley, 1983). We need to understand that women can have complicated feelings, including joy over the arrival of their babies and distaste for the birth experience itself.

Research examining the relationship between negative birth experiences and postpartum depression has yielded contradictory findings. Some researchers have found that use of obstetrical interventions is related to depression (Oakley, 1983; Thirkettle & Knight, 1985), while others have not (Chalmers & Chalmers, 1986; Cox et al., 1982; Knight & Thirkettle, 1987). Similarly, some researchers have found a relationship between obstetrical complications and depression (Davidson, 1972; O'Hara et al., 1984), while others have not (O'Hara, 1986; Paykel et al., 1980; Whiffen, 1988). One possible explanation for these contradictory findings is that the focus of these past studies was on objective complications or circumstances of birth rather than on women's subjective reactions to these events. This focus could be due in part to lack of a conceptual model of aspects of birth that create traumatic reactions. In this chapter we develop such a conceptual model and relate it to past findings.

CHARACTERISTICS OF TRAUMATIC BIRTHS

In this section we describe a conceptual model for negative birth experiences. This model is not meant to substitute for diagnostic criteria. Rather it provides a way of understanding women's experiences. The experiences of women reported in the literature and of women interviewed for this book vary widely. In some cases the behavior of the doctors or hospital staff was related to the negative reactions. In other cases the medical management was excellent but the circumstances of the birth (e.g., sudden complications or illness) were the problem.

We describe negative birth experiences in terms of traumatic stress, using Finkelhor's (1987) traumagenics model. The *traumagenics model* expands on the standard model of posttraumatic stress disorder (PTSD) by including interpersonal factors (such as the relationship between doctor and patient), which are important for understanding the full range of reactions to birth. According to this model, women might be affected by one factor or a combination of factors; the model does not assume that trauma is caused by the same events for everyone.

This model was developed originally to describe reactions to child sexual abuse. To adapt the model to birth experiences, we reviewed the qualitative and empirical literature on reactions to birth and found four dynamics related to negative or traumatic birth experiences: physical damage, stigmatization, betrayal, and powerlessness. Each of these is described below.

Physical Damage

For some women surgical incisions or other types of complications (e.g., hemorrhage, fractured coccyx, lower back injuries, and infections) can cause psychological trauma (Wessel, 1983). These physical symptoms in and of themselves are not necessarily trauma producing. The distinguishing characteristic is the woman's *interpretation* of the injuries: If she feels wounded or damaged by her experience, then these symptoms are trauma producing (Marut & Mercer, 1979). Even normal body changes such as lochia, leaking breasts, a flabby abdomen, and suddenly very obvious stretch marks can contribute to this feeling (Kitzinger, 1975). Some women have felt "mutilated" following their cesarean sections (Goer, 1991). In a survey of 228 women (Erb et al., 1983), 25%-30% of women having their first cesarean delivery expressed concern about their scars. And in a qualitative study, women with postpartum infections had more negative perceptions of their birth experiences than did women without infections (Tilden & Lipson, 1981).

Damage to the perineum also can be troubling. In her literature review, Oakley (1983) noted that 15%-37% of women surveyed who had had either episiotomies or episiotomies with perineal lacerations reported that their perineum was either "painful" or "very painful" at the end of the first postpartum week. Further, women who had had episiotomies experienced the highest percentage of breast-feeding difficulties. Even when women cognitively know that their perineum has healed, they might still feel "ruined" (Wessel, 1983). Others might be afraid of problems that could stem from perineal wounds, such as incontinence, perineal pain, and painful intercourse, or that their wound will "split open" from defecation (Kitzinger, 1975, 1987). Physical scars and painful complications also can traumatize women by reminding them of other trauma-producing aspects of their birth experiences. DeeDee, a pediatric nurse, describes how her ongoing complications, which required three postpartum surgeries to repair, were continual reminders of her traumatic birth experience:

> I had a traumatic delivery. . . . I had an epidural at 2:30 . . . and by 5:00 was fully dilated. I was told to push. I couldn't feel anything. I pushed for 2 hours and 15 minutes, but the baby's head wouldn't turn. I let the epidural wear off so I could feel. They had to use forceps. . . . They pulled the baby out in 15 minutes. They didn't wait for the epidural to start up again. The pain was *unbelievable*. I bent the bar on the table. I couldn't imagine that it would be that bad. I know I screamed. I felt really traumatized by it. After they pulled the baby out, I was just crying, but not from joy. I felt guilty about it. I didn't want to hold the baby. . . .
>
> I had granulation from the episiotomy. After 6 months, it abscessed. I went to see a surgeon. Where I had my episiotomy and tore, it was all infected and a mess. She cut out all that material.

Two weeks later, she said she might have to do surgery again. That's when the postpartum depression hit again. . . .
    My sister-in-law had a c-section. She's still disappointed that she didn't have a vaginal birth. I think she's crazy! She has *no* idea. I didn't say that to her, but at least you don't have the hemorrhoids or your tear doesn't hurt, and at least it doesn't hurt when you have sex. I've had sex maybe 10 times in the last year.

Stigmatization

The next dynamic described in the traumagenics model is stigmatization. *Stigmatization* occurs when a woman feels different from others because of some aspect of her birth experience or embarrassed by events that occurred during her labor and delivery (Balchin, 1975; Shearer, 1989). Mothers may feel shame or embarrassment if they feel that they lost control, if they screamed, swore, or had bowel and bladder accidents. Barbara describes her sense of shame following her labor:

My husband was embarrassed by noises I was making during delivery. He was telling me to be quiet. In a way, I feel like a failure because I took medication. I couldn't take it [pain] anymore. I think that has a lot to do with it. The back labor was excruciating.

Women may be embarrassed that a group of strangers saw them naked. Although many women may be embarrassed by these events, they are not necessarily traumatized. For others these elements may be traumatizing or may add to other traumatic elements of the experience. Wertz and Wertz (1989) recounted how many women felt that their most private parts were on display to the world, as this woman vividly describes:

What about the nameless parade of "interns" who appear unannounced, probe our trapped bodies and "scan" our progress? . . . I reached the point where I wouldn't have been surprised if the man who was washing the windows had suddenly laid down the sponge and come over to "take a peek." It seemed that everyone connected with the hospital was doing it! (p. 172)

Another possible source of stigmatization is from reactions of others when women describe their negative birth experiences.

Some women may feel as if they are the "only" ones who did not have a glorious birth experience. People around such a woman may tell her to "stop complaining," because she had a healthy baby. Some might deride her for being "selfish" or "ungrateful." Still others may tell her that all her pain was "worth it." Such comments as these completely invalidate a woman's experience and can make her feel as if something is wrong with her—why does she need all this special attention? It is important for women in these circumstances to recognize that they have a right to their responses. These women need support from people who will validate their experiences and help in their healing. This will do much to lessen the impact of their sense of stigmatization (Soloman, 1986).

Betrayal

The third dynamic in the traumagenics model is betrayal. This dynamic can be particularly acute for mothers who were interested and involved in their pregnancies and who made careful decisions about their deliveries (Tilden & Lipson, 1981). Women who expected to have a "natural" delivery and who were met instead with instruments, monitors, and obstetrical interventions feel particularly betrayed (Kitzinger, 1987; Ogier, 1982). Karen, who delivered with a nurse-midwife, describes her sense of disappointment and betrayal. During her 48-hour labor, she received numerous interventions, whose purposes were never adequately explained. She still feels ambivalent about her experience because she realizes that it could have been worse:

> I had all these expectations about what it would be like to deliver with a midwife. I was really making a radical decision, at least in my family, to do this. . . . I didn't realize until a month ago that it was a negative experience. That really set me up for depression, trying to deceive myself. I blame myself for what happened. I was conditioned. The whole prenatal experience conditioned me. . . . I don't want to make trouble. I know I got the best care available.

Betrayal can occur also when the persons whom a mother relied on to provide her care, in fact, harmed her. This is what Janoff-Bulman (1985) described as *shattered assumptions* that victims of trauma must redefine as part of their healing. When women in labor expect the support of the hospital staff and their doctors and instead are treated with rudeness, insensitivity, or even brutality, it can shatter their assumptions about the way things are supposed to be—"hospitals are supposed to help people." In a survey of 105 women who had cesarean sections (Affonso & Stichler, 1978), 31% of the women specifically cited the painfully rough and cold preparation for surgery. For Christine, a nurse who worked in the hospital where she delivered, the way she was treated during her delivery shattered her assumptions about the way doctors were supposed to behave and the way her colleagues should treat her:

> I was nervous about anesthesia from previous bad experiences. I decided to have an epidural and it didn't take. They told me I'd feel pulling but no pain. I could feel my legs being frozen, but I couldn't feel anything else. I told the anesthesiologist and she just patted me on the head and said I was "fine." I could feel *everything*. They gave me Novocaine. I was strapped to the table, screaming. The nurse stood by and cried and looked on in disbelief. My husband wasn't allowed to be there. The doctor wouldn't even allow him to be in the room for internals. He was very rude. . . .
>
> It was a beautiful day outside, and they were all complaining, saying they would rather be golfing. When it was time to be stitched up, they were supposed to give me something to sleep. I turned around, and the anesthesiologist was packing up. I had no anesthesia for being stitched up. The doctor gave me Novocaine. I could feel them stapling me. I had been with patients while having cesareans, so I knew all the layers. I felt everything. I think being a nurse made it worse. People question whether it really happened. My sister-in-law told my mother that she thought I had imagined it. But I know I didn't. I think I have a high tolerance for pain. . . .
>
> Being a nurse, I expected different treatment. I didn't expect to be treated any better, but I wanted to be treated like a colleague, the way I would treat everyone. What I got was anything but.

A woman also can feel betrayed by her own body, especially if she had a cesarean section because of "failure to progress" or some other ambiguous category (Tilden & Lipson, 1981). Even in cases with serious complications of labor, women still might feel inadequate or that their bodies let them down. Tracy, who developed eclampsia, expresses this idea:

I have always been physically active, and so I really thought my body had betrayed me. I tried to eat correctly, got plenty of exercise, and was never sick. High blood pressure happened to people who didn't do those things. I blamed myself a lot. I was told that it was because of too much salt that all this happened, but I didn't eat that much salt. I felt a lot of confusion.

Betrayal also can take place when a woman turns to others for comfort following a traumatic experience and is treated with harshness or indifference. This is what Silver (1986) described as *sanctuary trauma.* Sanctuary trauma occurs when a survivor of a severe stressor next encounters what she expected to be a supportive, protective environment and discovers that it is not what she expected. One example is the crime victim with the hospital and police. If she is treated with harshness or indifference, she may experience a second trauma. Following a traumatic birth experience, a woman might turn to female relatives, her husband, friends, or members of the medical profession only to be told to "pull yourself together." She might be greeted with outright hostility for her reactions (Dix, 1985). Elizabeth had her first panic attack following a negative birth experience while still in the hospital. She describes the reactions of people around her:

I tried to reach my doctor all night to no avail. My husband was very tired and didn't realize how important his support was to me. He told me to get some sleep and if I kept him up, he'd need to leave and go home to get some sleep. The doctor finally came in and didn't understand what was happening. I asked to see a psychiatrist before I left the hospital. She was very cool and not supportive. . . . The psychiatrist was very non-nurturant: not understanding, not available. She was curt on the phone when I called her for counseling. I had no help from these two women [the psychiatrist and her gynecologist]. For the next 2 weeks I was in constant panic.

These negative reactions of trusted individuals can cause trauma as surely as the birth experience itself (Chalmers & Chalmers, 1986). Because of the victim's vulnerability at this point, sanctuary trauma can be devastating and should be considered in any intervention that deals with the initial trauma.

According to Finkelhor (1987), the depression that follows a traumatic event could be a result of loss of a trusted figure.

These women may feel intense sadness at having lost someone they thought they could count on, both during their birth experience and afterward. Anger may follow these feelings of sadness and might be a way to protect against future betrayal.

Powerlessness

Powerlessness and the lack of control over labor and delivery are perhaps the key dynamics behind birth-related psychological trauma (Affonso & Stichler, 1978; Kitzinger, 1975). The importance of power and control is echoed over and over again in birth stories and in books preparing women for childbirth. Yet power is often the very thing laboring women lack (Kitzinger, 1987).

Control of birth experiences is one of the most consistent predictors of whether women will feel positively about them (Cranley, Hedahl, & Pegg, 1983; Tilden & Lipson, 1981; Trowell, 1982). In fact, in a study of women's reactions to cesarean sections, women's feelings of control have been correlated highly with their confidence during labor and delivery, their ability to relax during labor and delivery, successful use of breathing techniques, and how pleased they were with their deliveries (Marut & Mercer, 1979). Powerlessness also can diminish a woman's capacity to resolve her birth experience (Affonso & Stichler, 1978), and locus of control has been identified as a central dynamic in qualitative research examining women's reactions to cesarean birth (Tilden & Lipson, 1981). The loss of control caused by preparation for surgery caused severe anxiety for some of the women in their sample.

Because control and power are such important elements in determining whether a woman will have a negative birth experience, it is ironic that many hospitals specifically socialize women into powerlessness (Rothman, 1982; Wertz & Wertz, 1989). Hospital deliveries, by their very nature, have many aspects that make women vulnerable. Women are stripped of their clothing and are surrounded by strangers. Other people control their most basic functions, including when and what they eat and drink, whether they receive pain medication, and whether they can have a support person with them. They are likely to be subjected to a series of internal examinations and may be afraid to object for fear of being labeled a "bad patient."

Decisions about obstetric interventions are usually made without their input, and they often have little say about when they leave the hospital (Kitzinger, 1975; Shell, 1990). Many are simply informed that, ready or not, they will be discharged, as Barbara describes:

> I lost a lot of blood, my blood pressure dropped to 80/60. I couldn't nurse. They took the baby. I'd lift my head and throw up. They shoved me out in 3 days. My mom knew something was wrong. I couldn't stand without passing out. The doctor said "You're fine. Go home."

Elizabeth describes how the social environment of the hospital contributed to her psychic distress and physical pain:

> I had 25 hours of labor. It was long and hard. I was in a city hospital. It was a dirty, unfriendly, and hostile environment. There was urine on the floor of the bathroom in the labor room. There were 100 babies born that day. I had to wait 8 hours to get into a hospital room post-delivery. . . . There were 10-15 women in the post-delivery room waiting for a hospital room, all moaning, with our beds being bumped into each other by the nursing staff. I was taking Demerol for the pain. I had a major episiotomy. I was overwhelmed by it all and in a lot of pain. I couldn't urinate. They kept catheterizing me. My fifth catheterization was really painful. I had lots of swelling and anxiety because I couldn't urinate. My wedding ring was stuck on my finger from my swelling. The night nurse said she'd had patients that had body swelling due to not urinating and their organs had "exploded." Therefore she catheterized me again. They left the catheter in for an hour and a half. There was lots of pain. My bladder was empty but they wouldn't believe me. I went to sleep and woke up in a panic attack. I couldn't breathe and I couldn't understand what had happened.

The powerlessness dynamic has been described for other victims of a wide variety of traumatic events. According to Figley (1986), events are troubling to the extent that they are sudden, dangerous, and overwhelming. *Suddenness* occurs when an event strikes and there is no time to prepare, to devise an escape plan, or to prevent the event. This certainly occurs when women are in the hospital and in labor; they have no choice but to proceed. For example, in Affonso and Stichler's (1978) survey, 41% of the women had 2 hours or less to prepare themselves for their cesareans. Many procedures occur in rapid succession before a woman has time to process them, a rapidity that can lead to a feeling of sensory overload (Affonso, 1977). An emergency cesarean, especially, often catches women off guard and presents them with a drastic change in events (Cranley et al., 1983; Garel, Lelong, & Kaminski, 1987), as Christine describes:

> The second doctor decided within 2 hours to do a cesarean. He came and announced that he had decided this after he had already called the team to do a cesarean. We didn't necessarily agree. The doctor said, "If anything happens to your baby, it's your problem. I have people coming in, and I want to do a cesarean at 12. If you don't want to do it that way, it's your problem."

The *dangerousness* of the situation is the second element. Many women perceive that their labor or delivery is life threatening (Affonso & Stichler, 1978). In one study of cesarean section, women perceived the rush to the operating room as a "prelude to death" for them and their infants (Marut & Mercer, 1979). Fear of death leaves an imprint on the memory of all who experience it and certainly can contribute to trauma (Figley, 1986). Women in Affonso and Stichler's study reported fear from a variety of sources, including fear of death for themselves or their babies, fear of surgery, and fear of pain.

The final element is the extent to which the situation is *overwhelming*. Some women describe being swept away by their birth experiences and the hospital routines. Being overwhelmed leads to a sense of temporary helplessness and of being out of control. Affonso (1977) noted that the phenomenon of *missing pieces* (when women cannot remember important aspects of their birth experiences) is likely to occur when women have long labors with minimal information given to them about their progress or have rapid labors where they do not have time to process the events. In either of these cases, the women are overwhelmed by what is happening and are cut off from important information. Sally's emergency cesarean had all three aspects that are likely to put women at risk for traumatic stress reactions. Her baby was born within 15 minutes of when the cord prolapsed after she had been in labor for 23 hours:

> They had me on the bed, rear end in the air. My head was down between the headboard and the mattress. The nurse had to hold

the baby off the cord. All I kept hearing was "OB emergency, OB emergency" over the loud speaker, while the nurse kept saying in my ear that the baby would be fine. Everything happened so quickly, I didn't have time to react.

The above discussion focused on birth experiences in general. Now we turn our discussion to a form of birth that has been the focus of the majority of research on negative birth experiences: cesarean sections.

CESAREAN SECTIONS: DO THEY ALWAYS CAUSE PSYCHOLOGICAL TRAUMA?

Natural childbirth, I didn't really care about that. I was prepared to have an epidural. I didn't expect it to be life threatening. I was glad for the c-section. It saved my life. I don't resent it. It was more everything else [the medical complications; Kathy].

The majority of research on negative birth experiences has been on women's reactions to cesarean sections. Therefore this literature is worthy of a separate review. These studies generally have compared the experiences of relatively small samples (e.g., 20-40) of primiparous women who were delivered either vaginally or via emergency cesareans. The major findings are summarized below.

In one widely cited study, Marut and Mercer (1979) found that women who delivered via emergency cesareans had significantly worse perceptions of their birth experiences than did women who delivered vaginally. A number of factors predicted women's reactions to their deliveries. These included women's perceived sense of control during labor and delivery, fear during labor, worry about the baby's condition, time elapsed between delivery and prolonged mother-infant contact, type of anesthesia used (regional vs. general), and the presence of a support person during delivery.

Many of the findings of Marut and Mercer (1979) have been replicated in other studies. Women who had emergency cesareans had more negative perceptions of their births than did women who delivered vaginally (Bradley, Ross, & Warnyca, 1983; Cranley et al., 1983; Garel et al., 1987; Padawer, Fagan, Janoff-Bulman, Strickland, & Chorowski, 1988; Trowell, 1982) or women who delivered via planned cesareans (Cranley et al., 1983; Garel et al., 1987). Women who had regional rather than general anesthesia (Cranley et al., 1983; Garel et al., 1987; Padawer et al., 1988; Tilden & Lipson, 1981), who had a support person present during delivery (Cranley et al., 1983; Garel et al., 1987; Tilden & Lipson, 1981), and who had greater input in the decision-making process (Cranley et al., 1983; Garel et al., 1987) had more positive experiences than women who did not. Sally and Tracy, who both had emergency cesareans under general anesthesia, describe their reactions:

> We had made all the plans for natural childbirth. I wanted to avoid as much intervention as possible. I thought "I *will* do this. I can take it!" Nothing worked out as we had planned. . . . My husband wasn't able to be there either since they had to go in so fast. . . . I feel like I haven't even had a baby. I have no memory of it. I wish someone had taken a picture or video of the c-section. It just doesn't seem real to me [Sally].

> The birthing process was not a positive one for me. Everything my husband and I planned for and expected didn't happen. The hardest thing was having to be unconscious for the birth and my husband not being able to be there [Tracy].

Considering the importance of a support person being present, it is encouraging to learn that as of 1984, 80% of hospitals surveyed were allowing fathers to be present for cesarean births (Shearer, Shiono, & Rhoads, 1988), although many are still not allowed to be present for emergency cesareans under general anesthesia.

Mode of delivery also influenced whether women breast-fed their infants. Significantly fewer of the women who had had cesareans were breast-feeding (Bradley et al., 1983; Cranley et al., 1983; Trowell, 1982), with the lowest rate being for those who were delivered via emergency cesareans (Cranley et al., 1983; Trowell, 1982). On the other hand, Garel et al. (1987) found no significant difference in the percentage of women who were breast-feeding related to type of delivery.

On the positive side, three studies found no significant differences in reactions of women who had cesareans as compared with those who had vaginal deliveries. One study found no difference related to mode of delivery for marital adjustment, depression, or patterns of relating to their infants (Culp &

Osofsky, 1989). The authors explained their findings by describing their sample as well educated and middle class. The couples were said to be satisfied with their marital relationships before the baby and perhaps had been able to support each other through their cesarean sections. The authors also speculated that as cesareans become more common, less stigma is attached to them.

The other two studies found no differences in anxiety, depression, or how women related to their babies (Bradley et al., 1983; Padawer et al., 1988), based on mode of delivery. In fact, women in the cesarean group felt more confidence in their ability to mother (Bradley et al., 1983). The authors of both studies explained their findings by describing the particular environments of their hospitals or perinatal programs. Both studies were conducted in environments that specifically and systematically emphasized education of new parents and believed in follow-up postpartum care. The authors felt that these types of interventions prevented mothers from feeling bad about their birth experiences, provided a great deal of social support, and prevented any subsequent difficulties.

One longitudinal study (Trowell, 1982, 1983) comparing women who delivered via emergency cesarean sections ($N = 16$) and women who delivered vaginally ($N = 18$) had findings that contradicted the positive results of the three previously presented studies. This study found that women who delivered via emergency cesarean were significantly more depressed and anxious and had significantly less eye contact with their infants at 1 month postpartum than did mothers who delivered vaginally. At 1 year postpartum, the cesarean group reported having more difficulties with their infants, expressed more dissatisfaction and resentment at the demands made on them, and left their infants to cry longer (some waiting up to 5 minutes) than did the vaginally delivered group. At 3 years postpartum, mothers who delivered via cesarean sections were significantly more likely to report serious relationship problems with their children and were less likely to have completed their children's vaccinations than were mothers who delivered vaginally. This study demonstrates the long-lasting effects of negative birth experiences. It is important to note, however, that all the cesareans in this study were performed under general anesthesia, a factor shown to be related to negative reactions.

The mothers we interviewed who had general anesthesia all indicated that it had been difficult to bond with their babies because of their birth experiences. Kathy had eclampsia and was unconscious for 3 days after renal and liver failure, HELLP syndrome (Hemolytic anemia, Elevated Liver enzyme, Low Platelet count), and cerebral edema:

> I don't remember any of Sunday. . . . Sunday night I had the seizures and from this point on I was out. I was in something above a comatose state, but I was unconscious. I woke up Wednesday and found out I had a baby girl. . . . I knew I had a baby, but it didn't make sense. I couldn't take care of her. The last thing on my mind was my baby. I was thinking more of myself. One saving grace was being able to nurse. The nurses helped and held her on me. . . . Sometimes I still feel like she's not really mine, that someone else could take her away, that I don't have the right to make decisions about how to take care of her. Some of that response is because of low self-esteem because I didn't have a normal, healthy delivery. I'm afraid to give up nursing because it is the only tie that makes her mine, even though I'm getting pressure to give it up.

Tracy also had eclampsia and renal failure and had a similar response to bonding with her baby:

> I didn't get to hold my baby for over 16 hours. I only saw her once during that time. I feel the bonding has been long and hard. I wonder sometimes if some of it had to do with not seeing her or holding her for so long. It was over a day before I even held her for the first time.

Sally's reaction following her cesarean section for a prolapsed cord was also similar:

> It's taken a long time to bond with my baby. I haven't had any of the "new mother" euphoria people talk about. I did not get to hold my daughter until 8:30 the next morning. I let the nurses take care of her. I just wasn't up to it. I didn't even change a diaper until I went home. It's still hard for me to think of myself as a mother, sometimes.

In summary, the results of the above-cited studies indicate that cesarean sections can cause negative reactions for women who experience them and can influence how women respond to their babies. Certain aspects of cesarean delivery, including general anesthesia, absence of a support person, and an emergency cesarean, can make women more likely to respond negatively. These variations in responses also indicate that it is not the procedure of cesarean delivery per se that causes psychological trauma. As the results of three studies indicate, women who received ample support following their cesareans and who felt they had input in the decision-making process were significantly less likely to have negative reactions. Therefore cesarean sections do not have to be traumatic if women are provided with support and reassurance and are involved in decisions that concern them.

PROCESSING OF TRAUMATIC EVENTS

To help women who may have experienced a traumatic birth, it is important to understand how people process psychological trauma and what types of symptoms this processing might include. In this section we use a stress response model to describe women's reactions following a traumatic birth experience (Horowitz & Kaltreider, 1979). According to this model, people processing traumatic events proceed through a series of stages as they attempt to integrate the event into their cognitive framework. After the initial outcry, people oscillate between denial of the event and intrusive thoughts about it. The final stage is working through the trauma and attempting to find meaning in the event (Smith, 1986).

For persons processing trauma, the most prominent stages are denial and intrusive thoughts. Some of the characteristics of the *denial phase* include avoidance of anything connected with the event, numbness, reduced level of response to people or important activities, rigidly role-adherent or stereotyped behaviors, memory failure, and inattention or daze (Figley, 1986; Horowitz & Kaltreider, 1979). (Note that many of these symptoms are also classic symptoms of postpartum depression.) Some of these characteristics also might contribute to depression by increasing isolation and by having women set standards of perfection for themselves so high that they are doomed to failure, such as being the perfect mother after they "failed" in their deliveries. Denial also might explain why women who may have been traumatized by birth appear to be asymptomatic in the immediate postpartum period (Padawer et al., 1988) and why birth trauma may take weeks or months to emerge (Kitzinger, 1987; Marut & Mercer, 1979). *Intrusiveness* is manifested through reenactments of the event. Reenactments may be cognitive (as in flashbacks and intrusive thoughts) or physical (women put themselves in situations where they can reenact the event; Wilson & Zigelbaum, 1986). For example, some women purposely may seek to become pregnant again right away so that they can "do it right this time." Intrusiveness also is characterized by several other classic symptoms of postpartum depression, including hypervigilance, sleep and dream disorders, inability to concentrate on other topics, preoccupation with the baby or the birth experience, and confusion and disorganization.

The symptoms listed above have been cited not only for traumatic events in general but also for birth experiences specifically. For example, Affonso and Arizmendi (1986) described how women who have frequent and recurrent thoughts about their labors and deliveries are less likely to make a successful postpartum adjustment. Similarly, in an exploratory study of 85 women's reactions to their vaginal births, 86% reported that they could not remember parts of their labors or deliveries. Women experiencing this "missing-pieces" phenomenon have not integrated their experiences into their perceptions of the world. Behavioral manifestations of this lack include asking people the same questions over and over, having recurring dreams with birth-related themes, and being preoccupied with the past to the extent that they cannot focus on the present. This preoccupation can manifest itself as lack of interest in caring for the baby or showing signs of poor mother-infant interaction (Affonso, 1977). The connection between a negative birth experience and a lack of interest in the baby has been noted by others as well (Klein, 1990; Trowell, 1982). Women also reported dissociative reactions or having altered perceptions of their bodies during their cesarean sections, including feeling detached from their bodies or "spaced-out," having an altered time frame, or feeling as if they were watching from a distance (Affonso & Stichler, 1978). Kathy describes her experience following her near-fatal birth experience:

> I was learning every day how serious [my condition] had been. On top of it, a c-section. But things got better physically. Then I started

not sleeping in the hospital. At one point, the second week in the hospital was when it got scary. I realized I almost died. I felt so bad I didn't think I'd make it. It really hit then. Still nothing made sense. I didn't know if I was going to make it. I was still recovering from the water on the brain.

The depression hit 3 or 4 months later. Who knows what my body did to my hormones? My body was chemically completely haywire. The OB thought it was my brush with mortality. I honestly don't think that's it. I don't dwell on it because I didn't really see it; I was unconscious most of the time. . . . One area I still haven't worked through is the aloneness feeling it left with me. I felt very alone in the experience even though I had support. Death was knocking on my door alone. I also saw the world going on without me. These have probably been the hardest lessons I've learned and I'm still dealing with them.

Paradoxically, although some women may be preoccupied with their birth experiences, others may avoid activities or places that remind them of their traumatic experiences. For example, they may fail to show up for their postpartum checkup. Failing to show up for this checkup is also an important symptom of postpartum depression that is often ignored or misunderstood (Hotchner, 1988). Finally, women in the intrusive-thoughts phase may experience an increase in the intensity of symptoms when they are exposed to stimuli related to the event, including the hospital, their doctors, pregnant women, or other stimuli that remind them of the event. Elizabeth is still troubled by situations that remind her of the hot, stuffy environment of the hospital:

I still have problems sometimes, like when I'm on a hot bus in the summer. It reminds me of the hospital. . . . I've become claustrophobic, like when I'm on airplanes. It's the same thing, being out of control, hot and anxious.

Women who have had traumatic birth experiences must acknowledge their trauma if they are ever to move past it. Trying to "just forget it" is not an effective strategy, and trauma that is not acknowledged and dealt with will manifest itself in a variety of destructive and negative behaviors. Women who have not processed their trauma may manifest such symptoms as depression, blunted affect and inability to empathize with others (including their infants), helplessness, self-destructive behaviors, somatic complaints, sexual dysfunctions, marital difficulties, anger, and hostility. They also may become pregnant again before they are physically and emotionally ready to do so. Working through trauma is difficult, but it is the only route to healing. As a result of working through trauma, a woman has acknowledged and given herself permission to feel pain and anger following her experience. She may need a period of time to grieve over her experience. As trauma and grief are reclaimed, she can give meaning to the events and can move forward (Lindy, 1986). She even may come to value her experience and try to do something to help other people. This is what one article (Wilson & Zigelbaum, 1986) described as the "healthiest" form of coping with psychological trauma and was specifically mentioned by nearly all the women in this chapter who describe a negative birth experience.

In conclusion, the message from the research literature on recovery from traumatic events contains a message of hope: People can and do recover from psychological trauma. The most important components of any intervention focus on helping women acknowledge and accept their experiences and on helping them regain a sense of efficacy.

SUGGESTIONS FOR NURSES

Nurses can help women recover from negative birth experiences by being alert for possible symptoms of trauma, educating them about the process of trauma, and supporting them through their healing. In making these suggestions, we draw on nursing research dealing with cesarean sections and psychiatric literature dealing with posttraumatic stress disorder. Even though the majority of studies on negative birth experiences focus on cesarean sections, the suggestions for intervention also apply to negative reactions to vaginal births.

Preparing Women for the Unexpected

Whenever possible, women should be prepared psychologically for birth, including the possibility of cesarean section (Cranley et al., 1983; Marut & Mercer, 1979; Tilden & Lipson,

1981). This is an especially important suggestion for nurses who teach childbirth education, but it is also important for nurses who work with pregnant women in other capacities. This education helps minimize the psychological impact of unexpected events that occur during labor; such a reduction helps lessen their anxiety and helps them take part in decision making during labor.

Psychological Support During Labor and Delivery

As many of the women we spoke with indicated, the nurses often made the difference between a relatively good experience and a traumatic one. Standard obstetrical nursing texts offer a variety of suggestions on providing support during labor, delivery, and in the postpartum period. We limit our suggestions to types of activities that research studies have demonstrated are relevant to women's reactions to their birth experiences.

Strategies that nurses can employ include providing emotional support before and after labor (Tilden & Lipson, 1981), assessing and promoting relaxation and comfort, and providing information about what is happening throughout the course of labor (Affonso & Stichler, 1978). If the practitioner decides that a cesarean section, forceps delivery, or other type of intervention is necessary, nurses can help women cope by preparing them psychologically for the procedure (as should be done for all procedures) and by offering them emotional assurance. Further, these decisions should be discussed with the woman whenever possible. If at all possible, even in an emergency, a woman should be given the option of having her support person with her and of having regional anesthesia (Marut & Mercer, 1979), thus increasing her involvement in decisions regarding her care. Fathers also need to be informed about procedures rather than simply told to "leave the room."

Supporting the Woman in the Postpartum Period and Beyond

In the immediate postpartum period, it can be extremely helpful if a nurse reviews the woman's chart with her and answers any questions about what happened during labor and delivery. This dialogue helps fill in details about "missing pieces" and is especially important for women whose labors were very rapid, very long and drawn out, involved the use of medication (which could distort their perceptions), or for women who were delivered under general anesthesia (Affonso, 1977; Garel et al., 1987).

You also may talk with a woman after she has left the hospital or even months after her delivery. If you find that she is still troubled by aspects of her delivery (which is not unusual following a traumatic birth experience), encourage her to get her medical records and review them with her. In addition, if she has a positive relationship with her practitioner, encourage her to speak with him or her about her delivery as well.

Women in this situation may air feelings of anger, guilt, or disappointment. During this phase you can assist women by helping them place their experiences in a broader framework. This includes placing blame and credit more objectively (this is especially important when women are blaming themselves for what happened) and offering or supporting new and more generous or accurate perceptions of the event (Figley, 1986). Your intervention also may include making referrals to support groups for women who have had negative birth experiences or referring women to individual counselors (particularly those familiar with negative birth experiences and postpartum depression).

Intervention With Fathers

If you have the opportunity, you may need to intervene with fathers as well. Figley (1986) described how families can be traumatized vicariously by trauma of a family member. Two past studies (Erb et al., 1983; Stewart, 1985) found that fathers have reactions to cesarean sections similar to those of their wives, including anger and disappointment. It is reasonable to assume, given other research on posttraumatic stress reactions, that fathers would have similar reactions to their wives' negative vaginal birth experiences.

Fathers may need to deal with their feelings of having "failed" in their role as their wives' protectors and may not be able to support their wives adequately because of their own feelings of guilt and failure. They also may have to deal with their feelings of powerlessness in the hospital setting. Anecdotally, many fathers have reported feeling swept away by the hospital environment (e.g., McCormack, 1991). Helping fathers work through these feelings benefits them and their relationships with their families. It also may increase their participation in child care.

In the next chapter we examine the role of psychological and social factors in postpartum depression.

FOUR

Psychosocial Influences

After 3 weeks, I was afraid to be alone with my son. I was feeling completely inadequate as a mom. My mother-in-law was there looking over my shoulder and telling me what to do, telling me I wasn't giving him enough milk. She was bonding with him—I wasn't. I didn't have the emotional strength to fight for him back. She took over, thinking that was the right thing to do. Six weeks after he was born, I went back to work. This was really helpful. When I went back to work, the major anxiety and depression lifted. [Work] was something I knew I could do. When the colic stopped, that helped too [Elizabeth].

Psychosocial influences are a popular explanation for postpartum depression. People who do not attribute postpartum depression to "hormones" may attribute it to "unrealistic expectations" or "lack of support." Researchers also have paid a great deal of attention to psychosocial influences, and results of their studies have been remarkably consistent.

The *psychological factors* include a woman's worldview; her expectations about what it will be like to be a mother and how she will perform in her role; her self-esteem; how competent she feels as a parent; and prior vulnerability factors, such as previous psychiatric illness or a dysfunctional family history. The *social factors* include the amount of help she has with her baby and other children; the amount of emotional support she receives from her husband and others around her; demographic characteristics; and her exposure to stressful life events. Each of these is described in this chapter.

PSYCHOLOGICAL INFLUENCES

Attributional/Cognitive Style

I hadn't handled a lot of babies. The nurse was yelling at me saying, "What's the matter, haven't you handled a baby before?" I was offended and hurt. All I could think of was "I'm a bad mother." . . . When [the depression] was really bad, I thought, "I'm a bad person. I should have never had a baby, never gotten married. I'm a bad mother. I'm crap." I talked about it all the time until others were sick of hearing about it. . . . At one point my mom said to me, "I don't know what you are worried about. One baby is no work." All I could think was "I'm a failure" [Barbara].

How do people explain negative events in their lives? In everyday parlance we refer to people as either optimists or pessimists. Researchers use the more general term of *attributional style*. Attributional style predicts future vulnerability to depression following stress (Cutrona, 1983). According to the cognitive-vulnerability hypothesis, some people (the pessimists) have learned to interpret events in a way that makes them more stressful and negative. People with this attributional style see events as outside of their control and are more likely to experience learned helplessness (Manly et al., 1982). *Learned helplessness* leads people to believe that they cannot change negative aspects of their lives, and this attribution has been linked to depression in numerous studies (e.g., Cowan & Cowan, 1987). For example, the results of one large survey ($N = 809$) indicate that people who feel in control of at least some aspects of their lives have lower levels of depression. The authors speculated that people with some control are more likely to attempt to solve problems and to change their situations (Ross & Mirowsky, 1989).

In a reformulation of the learned helplessness model, Abramson, Seligman, and Teasdale (1978) identified three components of the helpless attributional style. Specifically, people with this cognitive style are more likely to become depressed after a negative event because they maintain internal, global, and stable attributions about why negative events occurred (Cutrona, 1983). *Internal* attributions mean the cause of the negative event is within the person's control either because of stable ("I am stupid.") or unstable ("I was tired.") characteristics. *Global* attributions mean the person feels that the negative event affects many areas of his or her life, while a person who makes specific attributions realizes that the negative event affects only one or two areas.

Although the research cited above refers to depression in general, attributional style also has been studied in relation to depression among new mothers. In two studies, negative attributional style during pregnancy was associated with postpartum depression at 2 to 3 months postpartum (Cutrona, 1983; O'Hara et al., 1982), and in one study it was not (Manly et al., 1982). Data were collected in the Manly et al. study at 3 days postpartum. Attributional style also predicted speed of recovery from postpartum depressive symptoms (Cutrona, 1983).

The authors of two recent studies (Donovan & Leavitt, 1989; Donovan, Leavitt, & Walsh, 1990) examined attributional style through a construct they referred to as *illusory control*. Subjects who had "high illusory control" were those who reported they have control over events that in reality were beyond their control. In a study of 66 mothers of 5-month-olds (Donovan et al., 1990), women with high illusory control were those who felt incompetent as parents and were more likely to withdraw from parenting situations. Many of these women experienced guilt when they could not be "perfect mothers." The authors speculated that this attributional style may lead to the overcontrolling and interfering behaviors that appear among depressed mothers of toddlers. In another study of 48 mothers of 5-month-olds (Donovan & Leavitt, 1989), women with high illusory control were the most depressed and reported the father as participating the least in child care activities. To summarize, women with the high illusory control attributional style were most susceptible to learned helplessness and subsequent depression. When they found they could not control the events they thought they could, they tended to give up and withdraw from the task.

Control appears to be a factor in both a positive and a negative attributional style. One way to understand these contradictory results is to examine how realistic these perceptions of control are. When people think they have no control over events that they can control (learned helplessness), or that they have control over events that are beyond their control (internal attributions for negative events), then they are likely to develop a pessimistic attributional style. The key appears to be learning to make realistic assessments about which events are controllable and which are beyond a person's control.

A preexisting negative attributional style may make women more prone to depression. A negative attributional style also can be caused by the stresses of childbearing. For example, a woman suddenly overwhelmed by depression may interpret subsequent events more negatively than she would have before the depression. Such interpretation can contribute to or aggravate the depression. Therefore it is possible for attributional style to be either a vulnerability factor or a by-product of depression. In either case it can contribute to depression. Researchers have concluded, however, that the explanatory power of attributional style tends to be small, especially when compared to other factors, such as life stress (Cutrona, 1983; Manly et al., 1982).

Self-Esteem, Self-Efficacy, and Expectations

All of a sudden I felt like I had to cook and freeze meals and sew—all the things I associated with being a mother. My husband kept saying to me, "But you've *never* liked to cook." I thought it was expected as a mother to do all these domestic things, even though I never did them before. . . . My house was pretty neat before, but I became obsessed with cleaning the house. Cleanliness of my house was important. I didn't want her to get a germ on her. . . . I thought I was the only one who could take care of my baby. I thought I'd never break free back into my other roles, which was ridiculous [Michelle].

Self-esteem, self-efficacy, and expectations are three concepts that refer to a woman's adjustment to her role as a mother, what she expects of herself, and how competent she feels as a parent. These concepts are closely related and tend to interact. According to Cutrona and Troutman (1986), those who have high self-esteem and a high perception of their own self-efficacy tend to be persistent, to avoid making internal attributions for their failures, and to experience less anxiety and depression. Those with low self-esteem and a low sense of self-efficacy tend to give up in the face of difficulties, to make internal attributions for their failures, and to experience high levels of both anxiety and depression. Expectations about what mothers are "supposed" to do influence how a woman evaluates the job she is doing and whether she will feel good about herself in her new role. In addition, unrealistic expectations of infants predicted depressive symptomatology in one study (Whiffen, 1988). Kathy found that it was very difficult to live up to what she perceived as others' expectations of her:

> The truth of the matter is that I'm ashamed. Why is it so hard for me and looks so easy for other mothers? I saw other full-time mothers always doing things better. I felt I couldn't keep up. I used to be able to "run with the guys." . . . Now, I'm in a traditional mommy role, but I'm not relating to this role. So where does this leave me? Not fitting into either role. . . . I'm used to being the best at what I do. But I felt I couldn't [function as a mother]. Especially when I look at other moms. I can't seem to understand why I can't do this. . . . I was depending on other people's expectations. Maybe even my own expectations were too high. This led to feeling down, out of control. That's when the depression really started. Doubting I could do it. It got to where I was scared to death, nervous, chest tightness, crying, not wanting to eat.

For DeeDee and Michelle, their nursing careers led to them placing unrealistic expectations on how well they would be able to handle their new babies:

> I'm a pediatric nurse. I thought it would prepare me to have a baby. It didn't. It's really different when it's your own baby.

> As a nurse, I thought I'd have this in-born knowledge of how to take care of a baby, even though I have always worked only with adults.

How competent a woman feels as a mother can influence whether she becomes depressed. In one study of 55 married women, parental self-efficacy acted as a mediator between infant temperament and postpartum depression. Women who had infants with difficult temperaments felt less competent as parents and had higher levels of postpartum depression. Social support buffered this effect by increasing self-efficacy and by helping the women feel more competent as parents (Cutrona & Troutman, 1986). In addition, maternal self-efficacy, as reflected in reports of feeling overwhelmed by child care, was associated with depression severity at 2 months postpartum (Campbell, Cohn, Flanagan, Popper, & Meyers, 1992).

Self-esteem also has been directly linked to postpartum depression. In a study of 80 postpartum women (Affonso & Arizmendi, 1986), a woman's view of herself and her future was significantly related to whether she was likely to be depressed. The key elements were "not feeling good about myself," "not managing roles well," "future does not look promising," "feel unattractive," and "predominant mood not positive." These items were all significantly and positively correlated with depression scores on the *Beck Depression Inventory* and the *Pitt Questionnaire* (a measure of postpartum depression).

A study of mothers of abused children also demonstrated a link between self-esteem, feelings of competence as parents, and depression in general (Kinard, 1990). The study compared mothers of abused children (*N* = 108) and a matched group of mothers of nonabused children (*N* = 108). The results revealed that the mothers of abused children had lower self-esteem, lower levels of support, and more negative perceptions of their competence as parents than did mothers of nonabused children. This result appeared even after controlling for maternal education and employment (two factors traditionally associated with depression; Ross & Mirowsky, 1989). In summary, women are more likely to experience postpartum depression if they have unrealistic expectations for themselves as mothers, if they have low self-esteem, and if they feel incompetent as parents. Social support appears to buffer these effects by increasing self-esteem and self-efficacy and by creating more realistic expectations.

Previous Psychiatric History/Prior Vulnerability

The final psychological factor is the psychiatric histories of women and members of their families. Previous psychiatric history has been found by a number of researchers to relate to postpartum depression. In one study (Paykel et al., 1980) this effect occurred independent of life events. Women with previous psychiatric diagnoses were significantly more likely to experience postpartum depression than were women with no such history. Watson, Elliot, Rugg, and Brough (1984) found that both psychiatric history of the subject and the subject's family were significantly related to whether she would experience postpartum illness. In addition, lability during pregnancy was associated with later postpartum disturbance for 128 women. Similarly, the number of previous depressions for the subject and depression among the subject's first-degree relatives were two significant vulnerability factors in a study of 99 postpartum women (O'Hara et al., 1984). More recently Campbell et al. (1992) found that a history of affective disorders for a mother or her first-degree relatives predicted depression severity at 2 months postpartum. Dawn had several relatives who experienced depression and psychosis:

> My maternal grandfather went through severe depression starting at the age of 35, right after his business burned down. From there on, he spent most of his life in various psychiatric hospitals. Shock treatment was necessary. My maternal grandmother went through postpartum depression after my mother was born. Later on in her life, she developed Parkinson's disease. I think her Parkinson's was caused by some of the medications she was on during her life. My mother suffered a psychosis depression [sic] during menopause. She still suffers from severe depression but without any psychotic episodes. Since menopause 4 years ago, she has been hospitalized about eight times. ECT treatments are usually necessary. My one brother used to have obsessive-compulsive disorder. He constantly washed his hands and was afraid of germs. Before pregnancy, I suffered from seasonal affective disorder, but I never had to be hospitalized.

Events that occurred during childhood are conceptually related to previous psychiatric history. Frommer and O'Shea (1973) found that women who had experienced childhood separation from their parents (either through death or divorce) were more vulnerable to postpartum depression than were their nonseparated counterparts. In a prospective study of 730 women, the mother's perception of maternal and paternal care during her childhood predicted postpartum depression (Gotlib, Whiffen, Wallace, & Mount, 1991). In contrast, a woman's loss of her mother or father did not predict postpartum depression in another study of 170 women (O'Hara et al., 1982). Watson et al. (1984) noted that some of their depressed subjects reported a connection between their current depression and a stressful past life event (e.g., loss of a parent). And McGrath et al. (1990) identified past sexual victimization as a major vulnerability factor in depression in general, although this has not been systematically explored with regard to postpartum depression. Three of the women interviewed for this book specifically indicated that their dysfunctional or abusive family of origin directly contributed to their depressions:

> I think childhood and personal history made a difference. My childhood was not unhappy, but I had an alcoholic father. I have had low self-esteem all my life. Not a lot of negative things, but very few *positive* things. I always pushed myself and was hard on myself. . . . I think a lot ties into childhood. My husband always expected that something would bring all of my childhood and teenage memories to a head [Michelle].

Elizabeth is concerned because of her mother's history of mental illness and substance abuse:

> My mom had had a nervous breakdown after the birth of my sister. I worried that that would happen to me. My mom is also a prescription drug addict. I worried about that too.

Val describes how her past history of sexual abuse related to her postpartum depression and how it manifested in obsessional thoughts of harming her twin babies:

> My depression started 3 days after birth. It came on very suddenly. My husband was coming to the hospital. We were going to give the babies a bath. As we were giving [my daughter] a bath, I was suddenly afraid that I might abuse her. I had been sexually abused as a child. I didn't tell anyone until the next day. . . . It started with, "Oh, my God. I was abused. I could abuse them." Then it was more general. Everything was a danger. Everything could hurt the kids. . . . I can't tell you how surprised I was. I haven't done anything to hurt the kids. I first visualized my son being thrown into the fire. Then it was me throwing him in. I worried about plastic. I'd have thoughts of smothering the kids with pillows. There were certain rooms in the house I couldn't even go in. I couldn't drink coffee. I'd have thoughts of pouring it on the kids. Through all of this I never neglected my children's needs, no matter how difficult. . . . No one ever questioned that I would hurt the kids. I'm the only one. I feel it could be from the sexual abuse. I obsess and worry about things. I've had times and traumatic events that I've worried about before, but it's always been just me. Now it's these kids that I want to take good care of. . . . My OB told me about another patient who couldn't take care of her kids for months. That was the worst thing he could say. . . . Something [else] that didn't help was when I called the DAD [Depression After

Delivery] support person in my state. She said she'd send some stuff. There was an article about women who killed their babies. I called another woman, and she told me about women who killed their babies. She said I had better take my thoughts seriously. Scary thoughts of hurting your baby are very common. This is important to know. They do not mean that you want to harm them. . . . I've felt so strange and weird through all of this. My doctors and therapist continue to reassure me that what I am feeling is "normal" for me [Val].

Sgroi and Bunk (1988) described the characteristics of adults who came in for treatment of childhood abuse and indicated that the precipitating factor for forcing the women (or men) to deal with these issues was often a stressful life event such as marriage or the birth of a child. It is therefore not surprising that a history of sexual abuse (or other dysfunctional family history) could precipitate postpartum depression. Research on family violence and the experiences of these women suggest that future research needs to expand its examination of previous psychiatric history to include psychiatric vulnerability caused by growing up in a dysfunctional home—even if the woman has never been diagnosed with a "psychiatric illness."

Summary

The above-cited studies demonstrate that how a woman feels about herself, her ability to control her environment, her certainty regarding her competency, her general outlook on life, and her family history can influence whether she will become depressed both in the puerperium and beyond. What these factors have in common is that they all occur within the woman herself. It is now time to turn our attention to aspects of her social environment and her relationships with others that can influence whether she will suffer from depression.

SOCIAL INFLUENCES

Social Support

This was the first grandchild on my side. I thought everyone would come to see me. My mom did, but only after I called and asked her to come. My dad came the next day, but only for the day. . . . I was very isolated after the baby. I had no friends with babies. It was hard. . . . I thought my family would come and everyone would hold the baby. Everyone came to my house at Christmas and they spent 6 hours in the basement playing video games. I was really hurt by that. Nobody would help me. I've really never said anything. Maybe it would have been better if I had said something [DeeDee].

A woman's level of social support is perhaps the single most important variable to consider in the study of postpartum depression. This variable examines her relationships with other people and the types of help she has available, especially in times of stress. Social support includes several types of assistance: instrumental, informational, and emotional support (Crockenberg, 1987). Lack of true social support is one of the best predictors of depression in general and postpartum depression (e.g., Kinard, 1990; O'Hara, Rehm, & Campbell, 1983; Ross & Mirowsky, 1989). Pregnancy and childbirth place increased demands on women, and the availability of social support is hypothesized as easing a woman's burden and increasing her ability to cope with the new demands. Karen describes how her sense of isolation increased her depression:

The pediatrician told me not to take her out for 6 weeks. I was housebound. Here I was, stuck in the house with a baby I couldn't stand. Before she was born, I kept thinking that having a baby would make everything wonderful. Afterward, I was terrified, thinking I shouldn't have had her. I told my husband I didn't want her. I was terribly depressed.

When considering whether a woman is receiving adequate support, it is easy to be fooled by appearances. We might assume that a woman who knows many people (has a large social network) or who is receiving assistance is experiencing social support (Howze & Kotch, 1984). But this is not always the case. For example, in one study of 170 women, the size of a woman's social network did not predict postpartum depression (O'Hara et al., 1982). People in a woman's social network might not offer to help. And even if they help, the woman must *perceive* it as support. Unwanted help can undermine a woman's confidence in her ability to perform her tasks as a mother, can threaten her self-esteem, and can engender dependency on the person providing the help. Even when a woman is grateful for the assistance, she may be uncomfortable accepting it if she is an independent or private person and is used to doing things for herself (Affleck, Tennen, Rowe, Roscher, & Walker, 1989). Christine describes how having her mother and her in-laws come to help after the baby was born made her uncomfortable:

> Everyone was really helping with the baby but me. They were *too* supportive. I know my husband wouldn't want to think that. I felt like they were taking over everything, that I had to be able to do it all. I kept trying to be the perfect wife. I'm a very private person. I felt like everything was exposed.

Researchers often examine relationships within a woman's immediate family and have found that husbands can be a key source of social support. In a study of 120 postpartum women, Paykel et al. (1980) found that depressed mothers reported significantly less emotional or instrumental support with children or household chores from their husbands than did the nondepressed mothers. Indeed the women's perception of their relationship with their husbands was significantly correlated with depression. These findings were confirmed in another study of 43 mothers of 13-month-olds (Levitt, Weber, & Clark, 1986). Although these women identified 13 people on average as being in their social networks, the primary source of support came from their husbands, followed by their own mothers. Lack of spousal support was an independent predictor of whether mothers would report negative affect and less life satisfaction. O'Hara (1986) also found that women experiencing depression reported both less instrumental and emotional support from their husbands than did their nondepressed counterparts. In a prospective study of 730 women, the depressed women reported lower marital satisfaction than did the nondepressed women (Gotlib et al., 1991). Another study of 128 postpartum women demonstrated that low levels of satisfaction with the marital relationship and low overall ratings of the marriage in general were related to higher levels of postpartum depression (Watson et al., 1984). A prospective study of 105 women (Cox et al., 1982) found that depressed subjects were more likely to report a deterioration of the marital relationship than were their nondepressed counterparts. Spouse's amount of help with child care and household tasks predicted depression severity at 2 months postpartum (Campbell et al., 1992). Further, spousal support interacted with pregnancy and delivery complications, so women with more complications and lower levels of support were more likely to be severely depressed. In this same study, women with less spousal support were also more likely to be chronically depressed, even up to 2 years later. Michelle describes how her husband was instrumental in her recovery:

> Support of my husband really helped. He never gave up on me. He's very, very strong.

Another aspect of social-support research involves the entire social network. Certain features of the network that are of interest to researchers include the total size of the network (number of people involved), number of confidants, proportion of kin, frequency of contact, and reciprocity in supportive interactions. O'Hara et al. (1983) examined these factors related to social networks, comparing a sample of depressed ($N = 11$) and nondepressed ($N = 19$) puerperal women. The results of that study revealed no significant difference in size of the social network and number of confidants for the two groups. In addition, proportion of kin in the social network was not significantly different. Interestingly, depressed subjects had more contact with their network than did their nondepressed counterparts. In spite of this increased level of contact, the depressed women reported receiving less emotional and instrumental support. The major differences between the groups appeared in the abilities of each at giving and receiving support. The depressed women reported that they *gave* less support to their spouses, parents, and confidants and *received* less emotional support from this same group. The authors hypothesized that perhaps this lower level of social support for the depressed women was an effect rather than a cause of the depression in that depressed people often become aversive to family and friends. In addition, friends or family may be uncomfortable dealing with someone who is depressed. Joanne describes this reaction from most of her friends but notes that one friend continued to reach out to her:

> I was usually an outgoing person, but I didn't have the energy to relate to others. My friends didn't know what to do. They thought

I had had a nervous breakdown. Many stayed away. Even now, many are surprised that I can still function. I had one friend who was very supportive and loving continually, even though she didn't understand. She brought meals, wrote little notes. She made no demands on my recovery. My mother-in-law and husband were helpful during that time too.

A study by Cutrona (1984) indicates that type of social support also has an influence. In her study of 71 primiparous women, overall level of support was only predictive of depression in the later weeks of the postpartum period. The two aspects of social support that were most predictive of depression were *social integration* (the network of people with whom the mother shares interests and concerns) and *reliable alliance* (people whom the mother can count on for help in any circumstance). Cutrona explained her findings about the linkages of social support to postpartum depression by noting that contact with others may have helped the woman problem-solve, led to her developing less threatening attributions about problems, provided opportunities for reinforcement from others, and increased her self-esteem and self-efficacy beliefs.

Social Structures

The above-cited studies focus on women's networks involving family or friends. Another type of social support research has examined the role of the culture in which women live. In an anthropological review of the literature, Stern and Kruckman (1983) found that the blues are virtually nonexistent in the cultures that they described and noted that these cultures all have (a) social structuring of postpartum events, (b) social recognition of a role transition for the new mother, and (c) instrumental assistance to the new mother. For example, in China and Nepal very little attention is paid to the pregnancy; all the attention is focused on the mother *after* the baby is born. The characteristics of this type of support are listed below.

A distinct postpartum period. In almost all the societies studied, the postpartum period is recognized as a time distinct from normal life. It is a time when the mother is supposed to recuperate, her activities are limited, and the woman is taken care of by her female relatives. This also was common practice in colonial America and was referred to as the "lying-in" period (Wertz & Wertz, 1989).

Protective measures reflecting the new mother's vulnerability. During the postpartum period new mothers are recognized as being especially vulnerable. In some cultures the postpartum period is considered to be a time of ritual uncleanness, while in others it is a time for the mother to rest, regain strength, and care for the baby.

Social seclusion and mandated rest. Related to the concepts of pollution and vulnerability are the widespread practices of social seclusion for new mothers. During this time she is supposed to rest and restrict normal activities. In the Punjab, a woman is secluded from everyone but female relatives and the midwife for 5 days. After the 5 days a "stepping out" ceremony takes place for the mother and baby. Seclusion is said to promote nursing, and it limits her normal activities.

Functional assistance. To make sure that women get the rest they need, they must be relieved of their normal workload. The personal assistance involves care of older children, household help, and personal attendance during labor. As in the colonial period in the United States, women often return to their families' homes to ensure that this type of assistance is available.

Social recognition of her new role and status. In cultures with a low incidence of the blues or depression, a great deal of personal attention is given to the mother. This has been described as "mothering the mother." In these various cultures the new status of the mother is recognized through social rituals and gifts. For example, the Punjabi culture has the ritual stepping out ceremony, ritual bathing and hair washing performed by the midwife, and a ceremonial meal prepared by a Brahmin. When the new mother returns to her husband's family, she returns with many gifts that she has been given for herself and the baby. Ritual bathing, washing of hair, massage, binding of the abdomen, and other types of personal care are also prominent in the postpartum rituals of rural Guatemalan women, Mayan women in the Yucatan, and Latina women both in the United States and Mexico.

Stern and Kruckman (1983) presented these structural differences in cultures as evidence contradicting the idea that the blues and depression are ubiquitous or inevitable (as has been described in some sources they cite). They concluded that the lack of documented incidence of mild postpartum depression in the cross-cultural literature, contrasted with the high incidence in the United States and other industrialized nations, suggests that this phenomenon is "culture bound."

Cox (1988), however, pointed out that it is naive and inaccurate to claim that postpartum illness does not occur in non-Western cultures. He reported on his research in East Africa and described how in these cultures, which also have elaborate social rituals associated with delivery, there appears to be incidence of both postpartum depression and psychosis. He concluded by stating that postpartum illness cannot be considered merely a cultural artifact.

The differences between the results of the two analyses perhaps are found in the definition of *social rituals*. In the Stern and Kruckman (1983) article, the social rituals involved providing some support for the mother. She was given personal attention and care and was relieved temporarily of her day-to-day duties. The rituals described by Cox (1988) focused on the legitimacy of the fetus. For example, an older woman was assigned to the pregnant woman to be sure that no taboos were violated that could call into question the legitimacy of her child (such as not allowing a man to step over her legs). A naked pregnant woman was examined by her husband's clan to ensure legitimacy of the child, and after birth the midwife determined legitimacy by seeing whether the umbilical cord floated when put into a mixture of beer, milk, and water. Any difficulties that a mother encountered during her labor were said to be a result of her own immorality. These rituals acted as tests of legitimacy and were not particularly supportive toward mothers. In fact they probably increased her stress level. (The author did not state what happened to babies who were determined to be illegitimate.) It appears that the *existence* of rituals is not enough to ensure that women do not suffer from postpartum illness. The *type* of rituals is also important. Rituals that appear to be effective in preventing postpartum illness are those that provide support and assistance for new mothers.

The lack of social structures following birth has been expressed by many new mothers. After a baby is born in our culture, all the attention shifts from the mother to the baby. One popular book written for new mothers (Eisenberg et al., 1989) describes this transition as "the reverse Cinderella—the pregnant princess has become the postpartum peasant" with a "wave of the obstetrician's wand" (p. 546). Many of the mothers interviewed for this book felt a profound sense of loss and abandonment by their medical caregivers and their families. In general there was little acknowledgment of what these women had been through, both physically and emotionally, by giving birth:

I really wanted someone to make me feel special. All the attention was on the baby [Barbara].

I feel a sense of anti-climax. I was used to being the center of attention. Then I had to go back to being a normal, healthy person. I'm not begging for attention, but now everyone only pays attention to the baby. It would be nice to have some attention afterward. While you're pregnant, you're feeling fat and slobby and don't want it. After the baby, you want it [Julie].

I felt like I didn't matter. I felt like they weren't interested in me after I had my baby. . . . My husband said, "Of course, they are not interested. You've had your baby." The 6-week visit seemed like an eternity away. I wrote [my midwife] a note to thank her. She didn't even mention it when I saw her at 6 weeks. . . . When I felt great, they treated me nicely. Now when I feel so awful with this baby, no one seems to be available to me [Karen].

My doctor thought her job was done after my daughter was born. It's ridiculous to think the job is done just because you've delivered the baby. I called her a couple of times after, and she told me to see a social worker. I eventually left my OB. There were many reasons, but mainly because she left me high and dry after delivery [Jan].

After the birth, I had several people tell me that the most important thing was that I had a healthy baby. Yes, that is important. But what about me? No one pays attention to the fact that you've had major surgery. They would have paid more attention if you had had your appendix out [Sally].

Rothman (1982), in her sociological analysis of American childbirth practices, described how pregnancy, birth, and the postpartum period are viewed as discrete events instead of different stages of the same process. This could account for some of the profound letdown that many women feel. Oakley (1983) pointed out that normal care of a newborn involves many activities that would be forbidden for days or even weeks following abdominal surgery but are expected of women following cesarean section. In the United States in particular, the "lying-in" period tends to end when the woman leaves the hospital (O'Hara, 1986), and women's length of hospitalization is becoming shorter all the time (Shell, 1990). A key to prevention of postpartum depression lies in continuation of the caregiving process through the end of the postpartum period and beyond.

Additional Benefits of Social Support

The focus of this section so far has been on the effect of social support in lowering levels of depression. Social support also can provide a number of other benefits to ease a woman into her new role and make her feel more confident. Social support provided by professionals (social workers) and nonprofessionals (experienced mothers who served as role models) significantly lowered levels of anxiety in highly anxious primiparous women (Barnett & Parker, 1985). In addition, high levels of social support benefit the mother-child relationship. Social support has been related to mothers being more sensitive to their infants in the first year (Crockenberg & McCluskey, 1986). This trend continued until the children were older. In a study of 38 mother-child dyads (with children ages 27-55 months), the more support a mother received in her role as a parent, the better were her interactions with her child. This result applied to mothers who were single parents, as well as to those who were in two-parent families (Weinraub & Wolf, 1987).

Conversely, lack of support from fathers predicted the high illusory control attribution style (Donovan & Leavitt, 1989), and perceived lack of support from fathers also was related to insecure attachments between 34 Japanese mothers and their 12-month-old infants (Durrett, Otaki, & Richards, 1984). The authors interpreted their findings by stating that mothers who did not have support may have had higher levels of stress, which made them psychologically unavailable to their infants. And lack of social support was also characteristic of mothers who neglected their children, even when controlling for the effects of socioeconomic status (Polansky, Gaudin, Ammons, & Davis, 1985). In general, mothers with high support are more satisfied with their babies, their maternal roles, and their lives overall (Crnic & Greenberg, 1987).

Life Events

In addition to social support, another outside influence is the number of stressful life events. In a study by O'Hara et al. (1983), the authors compared the number of stressful life events in the lives of depressed (N = 11) and nondepressed (N = 19) puerperal women. Consistent with their hypothesis, the depressed women had experienced more stressful life events since the beginning of their pregnancies than had the nondepressed women. An earlier study of 170 women had similar results (O'Hara et al., 1982). Another study of 120 women demonstrated that depressed women had experienced significantly more negative life events during every trimester and since the birth of their baby than did their nondepressed counterparts (Paykel et al., 1980). Similar results were reported in O'Hara's (1986) study of 99 women. And Watson et al. (1984) found relationships between depression and four distinct types of life events: (a) acute life events with no relation to pregnancy, (b) acute life events directly related to pregnancy, (c) general life difficulties, and (d) events that caused depression for these women in the past (e.g., death of a parent). All but 3 of 29 women who fit the criteria for "depressive neurosis" (out of a sample of 128) had experienced one of these types of life events. Dawn describes how several major life events occurred within 3 months of her giving birth and were related to her experience of both postpartum depression and psychosis. (Dawn also had a family history of depression, which was described in an earlier section).

[The first event was] a very traumatic labor and c-section. Two weeks after the birth, my father died suddenly from a heart attack. A week after my father's death, my mother went through another severe depression and had to be hospitalized for over a month. When my mother got out of the hospital, my grandfather (her father) died. This all happened during the winter, and as I mentioned before, I was suffering from SAD (seasonal affective disorder). I was also having financial problems and problems with my relationship with my boyfriend.

Women who were highly anxious in the puerperium reported more life events during their pregnancies, but they also reported more distress per life event (Barnett & Parker, 1985). The authors reported, however, that the main difference between the anxious and nonanxious groups was the perception of the events: The anxious group was more likely to perceive the events as being more negative and distressing. Prepartum life stress predicted depressive symptomatology in 115 primiparous women (Whiffen, 1988). O'Hara et al.'s (1984) study found no relation between depression and life events but did find significant relationships between other measures of life stress and depression, such as obstetric risk factors and child care stress. Overall, the authors of this study concluded that it is not the gradual accumulation of stressors that causes depression. Rather it is a series of stressors that occur over a fairly short time. Similarly, Cowan and Cowan (1987) observed that it is not the sheer amount of life stress that occurs that causes difficulties, but the balance between life stress and available support. When support is inadequate, stressful events have negative effects on young families. It appears that life events can act as stressors and are particularly likely to cause postpartum depression in the face of a prior vulnerability factor (such as negative attributional style), low self-esteem and self-efficacy, lack of social support, or a combination of these factors.

Demographic Characteristics

Research on the relationship between postpartum depression and variables such as maternal age, marital status, and parity has yielded inconsistent results. Few researchers even include these variables in their studies because the majority of studies have samples consisting primarily of married primiparous middle-class women. Nevertheless, a few studies have included subjects from more diverse backgrounds, thus allowing researchers to examine demographic characteristics. The following is a summary of these findings for age of the woman, parity, marital status, and socioeconomic status.

In one study, researchers found that age of the woman was related to depression, with the younger subjects being more likely to become depressed (Paykel et al., 1980). Other researchers

(Davidson, 1972; O'Hara et al., 1984; Watson et al., 1984) found no relationship between age and depression. The study of parity yielded similar type of findings. Davidson (1972) found that multiparity is related to higher incidence of the blues in Jamaican women (especially for women who had from 5 to 9 children). These women also were among the poorest in the sample, however. The author believed that low socioeconomic status (SES) could have contributed to higher incidence of the blues among multiparous women. In contrast, Ifabumuyi and Akindele (1985) found that primigravidae had higher incidence of psychosis than did multigravidae. And Watson et al. (1984) found no relationship between parity and depression.

Watson et al. (1984), Davidson (1972), and O'Hara et al. (1982) found no relationship between marital status and depression, and O'Hara et al. (1984) did not find a relationship between depression and number of years the woman was married. Marital status may have an indirect link to depression, however, through the mediators of stressful life events and lack of social support, with single parents more likely to experience both of these than are mothers in two-parent families (Weinraub & Wolf, 1987).

Surprisingly few researchers have examined the relationship between socioeconomic status and postpartum depression, despite the fact that poverty has been identified as a major risk factor for depression in general (McGrath et al., 1990). As with other demographic characteristics, the effects of SES have yielded inconsistent findings. The results of four recent studies indicate no relation between SES and depression (O'Hara et al., 1982, 1984, 1991; Watson et al., 1984). Researchers found, however, that depressed women were significantly more likely to report difficulties with housing (an issue related to SES) than were their nondepressed counterparts (Paykel et al., 1980). Finally Watson and Evans (1986) assessed three groups of new mothers in Great Britain: indigenous (English), Bengali, and "other" immigrants. The "other" group included West Indians, Vietnamese, Chinese, Egyptians, and Sikhs. The results of their study indicate that although depression appeared in all three groups, the problems continued past the first postpartum year for the poorer (immigrant) groups. The authors suggested the greater risk of depression continuing when there are ongoing problems in the women's lives.

The Watson and Evans (1986) study has important implications. First, it indicates that postpartum depression is not merely a middle-class phenomenon, because it occurs in low-SES women as well. Second, it indicates that low-SES mothers are at even greater risk for ongoing depression than are their middle-class counterparts. Community and family support for new mothers, however, can alleviate or prevent depression, even in poorer communities. Recall that many of the cultures described by Stern and Kruckman (1983) were in the Third World. Yet these cultures were often far more effective in supporting new mothers than were cultures with greater economic advantage. Similarly, Polansky et al. (1985) found that women who had connections with others in their communities were less depressed than were those who did not, and this occurred even in poorer neighborhoods. Therefore, as we have said previously, intervention for all mothers requires increasing their sense of social support within the community; this can be accomplished even in communities with few economic resources. (See U.S. Advisory Board on Child Abuse and Neglect [1991] for suggestions on creating supportive environments for new mothers.)

In summary, although research conducted with middle-class samples has yielded valuable information, it is now time for researchers to include a broader range of women in their studies. Including women from diverse backgrounds would enable researchers to apply their results to women in a variety of life circumstances.

Summary

Of the social factors considered, far and away the most influential is a woman's perception of her social support. As the research on nonpostpartum depression has repeatedly demonstrated, lack of social support is related to depression. This is especially true when women are faced with numerous negative life events within a short period of time—for example, stressful birth experience, birth of a handicapped baby, death of someone in her immediate family, or marital problems. Social support also is related to many of the psychological factors described above. Social support increases self-esteem and self-efficacy, acts a buffer when a woman is faced with a temperamentally difficult child, and even can alter a woman's attributional style. Therefore it becomes apparent that any effort to prevent postpartum depression must include a strong component aimed at increasing social support.

SUGGESTIONS FOR NURSES

Increasing Parenting Self-Efficacy

Women who are low in parenting self-efficacy are more likely to become depressed. Nurses can increase mothers' confidence by teaching basic parenting skills. This could include teaching mothers to read their babies' cues (especially important in dealing with a difficult or sick baby) and supporting women in their efforts to breast-feed. This type of education already takes place in most hospitals, but contact with mothers tends to be brief as hospital stays grow shorter. If you are not in a position to provide this type of education yourself because of time constraints or lack of ongoing contact with mothers, consider developing a list of other education resources in your community. If no resources exist, consider approaching your local hospital or parenting program about starting such a program.

Increasing Social Support

Social support is another key element related to depression. Nurses, particularly visiting nurses, can be extremely effective in this area. In one study (Holden et al., 1989) home-health nurses were given 6 hours of training in nondirective counseling techniques. They then visited mothers for 8 successive weeks and provided "therapeutic listening" and social support. The women who received this intervention ($N = 26$) were significantly less depressed than were the control women ($N = 24$). Of the women who received the home visits, 88% identified talking to the health visitor as the most important factor in their recovery.

The Holden et al. study demonstrated that nurses are very capable of providing this type of support but that many cannot because of time restrictions or the type of contact they have with mothers. Even if you are not in a position to provide this type of support, you can help by asking women very specific questions about how they are feeling, validating their experiences, helping them see that they deserve help and support, and working with them to get support from their husbands and other people in their social networks. Providing anticipatory guidance in the prenatal period can give mothers a head start in mobilizing their social resources. This might mean developing a list of community resources that will help her obtain ongoing support. Types of resources include support groups, places where she can meet other new mothers, postpartum care providers, and even people who provide practical assistance such as cleaning house or running errands. You also might need to develop a list of mental health professionals who are knowledgeable about postpartum illness and can help mothers long term.

Helping Women Overcome
Psychiatric Vulnerability to Depression

A final factor to consider is the woman's past history. As this chapter demonstrates, childbirth can bring up many conflicts or hurts from the past. Mothers might need referrals to mental health specialists or support groups that deal with issues such as physical or sexual abuse or adult children of alcoholics. For the most part these problems will be too involved for your average contact with mothers. But your recognition of the problem and your offer to provide a referral can encourage her to seek assistance on her own. She may feel too overwhelmed to seek out these resources for herself.

In the next chapter we examine the role of the infant in postpartum depression.

Infant Characteristics

My baby was very colicky. She had a reflux problem that lasted 5-6 months. In the beginning she had projectile vomiting. She threw up after every meal. I had overactive letdown, so she couldn't keep up with nursing. Our doctor was not understanding. . . . "Welcome to parenthood" or "You're stressed" is all he'd say. . . . I got to the point where I didn't want to touch her. I'd start to nurse and she'd scream [Barbara].

In the previous three chapters we focused on characteristics of the mother or of the mother's environment that contribute to her depression. This emphasis represents the state of the field itself. To date, the majority of studies on postpartum depression have focused on characteristics of mothers, and researchers have paid little attention to the effects of infants on the mothers' emotional state (Hopkins et al., 1984). This focus may be partly due to the tendency to view infants as passive participants in the mother-infant relationship. Infants were hypothesized as bringing little to the interaction (the *tabula rasa* or "blank slate" conceptualization), and mothers were considered to be responsible for their infants' behaviors (Campos, Bartlett, Lamb, Goldsmith, & Stenberg, 1983; Santrock & Yussen, 1992). Prior to the work of Lewis (Lewis & Lee-Painter, 1974) and Brazelton and colleagues (Brazelton, Tronick, Adamson, Als, & Wise, 1975), the influence of infant temperament on behavior was ignored, as was the reciprocal nature of mother-infant interactions.

More recently, researchers have acknowledged that the mother influences the child's behavior and that the child influences the mother's behavior (Macey, Harmon, & Easterbrooks, 1987; Rieser-Danner, Roggman, & Langlois, 1987; Santrock & Yussen, 1992). This is known as a *transactional* or *bidirectional approach*. The bidirectional approach also provides a framework for understanding the role of the infant in postpartum depression, focusing primarily on the effectiveness of the mother-infant relationship. An effective (or synchronous) mother-child interaction contains many components (Capuzzi, 1989). The mother and infant must give clear cues to each other, the mother must be responsive to the infant's cues, the infant must respond to the mother's caregiving, and the environment must be supportive of and facilitate this interaction. This is the process by which mothers become "attached" to their infants.[1] When this process breaks down, it can lead to insecure attachments between mothers and babies and to maternal depression.

In Chapter 4 we described psychosocial elements that might make women vulnerable to depression, and many of these characteristics relate to the mother-infant relationship. In this chapter we describe infant characteristics that can relate to depression. Specifically, we explore the psychological ramifications for mothers of infant temperament, infant illness, prematurity, or disability. We also describe the interplay between these infant characteristics and mothers' self-esteem, self-efficacy, and social support. Even though the primary focus of this chapter is infant characteristics, constant interaction occurs between the baby's and mother's characteristics.

INFANT TEMPERAMENT

As current research has indicated, babies bring their own personalities to their relationships with their mothers. Babies' personalities include how much they cry, how shy they are, how distractible, irritable, soothable, and active. This study of infant personality is more commonly known as the study of infant temperament. Broadly defined, *temperament* is a behavioral style and characteristic way of responding (Santrock & Yussen, 1992). Temperament is stable and describes dispositions rather than discrete behaviors (Campos et al., 1983).

Several researchers have explored and categorized the dimensions of infant temperament (e.g., Buss & Plomin, 1975;

Rothbart & Derryberry, 1981). The most commonly cited work on infant temperament, however, is that of Chess and Thomas (Chess & Thomas, 1977; Thomas & Chess, 1987). On the basis of their research, Chess and Thomas described infant temperament as falling into three basic types: easy, difficult, and slow-to-warm-up. An *easy child* tends to be in a positive mood, adapts easily to new experiences, and quickly establishes routines in infancy. A *difficult child* reacts negatively and cries frequently, is slow to accept new experiences, and does not engage in regular routines. A *slow-to-warm-up child* has a low level of activity, shows low adaptability, is somewhat negative, and displays a low intensity of mood. In their longitudinal study, Chess and Thomas (1977) classified 40% of the children as "easy," 10% as "difficult," and 15% as "slow-to-warm-up." The remaining 35% were somewhere between these three categories. Thomas and Chess (1987) conceptualized temperament as a stable characteristic of newborns that is later shaped and modified by the children's experiences.

The difficult child is central to our study of the infant's impact on postpartum depression. Difficult infants have strong emotional reactions; cry for long periods of time; are hard to comfort; are slow to accept new people, foods, or routines; and are less easy to predict or regulate in their eating, sleeping, or elimination schedules. These babies might be described as "colicky" by mothers and other people around them (Cutrona & Troutman, 1986; Rieser-Danner et al., 1987). In some cases temperament is assessed on the basis of the mother's perception of it (by asking her to rate how much the baby cries, etc.). In other cases more objective measures (such as Brazelton's Neonatal Behavioral Assessment Scale) are used to assess temperament. For purposes of this discussion, the mother's *perception* of temperament is more relevant because her perception of the infant is likely to influence her emotional state (regardless of what the "objective" measures state). In one study the mother's *subjective* reaction to her baby and her sense of control were better predictors of the severity of her depression than were measures of infant difficultness (Campbell et al., 1992). In addition, in many cases mother's perceptions and objective measures agree. Such was the case with Melissa, who describes her baby this way:

> My first baby screamed from the day he was born. He screamed all the time, even in the hospital. He reacted oddly to all kinds of

different things. The pediatrician said he was a "difficult" child. Even now, he has to have things always the same. . . . When I went back for a checkup at 2 weeks, a nurse asked me how the baby was. She said, "Aren't they wonderful?" I didn't know what to say. I thought he was the pits. I think people need to ask more questions instead of waiting for the woman to bring it up.

Dalton (1971) found that a significantly higher percentage of women who experienced the blues had a crying baby, a baby who vomited frequently, or a baby who was keeping the mother up at night. Another study (Cutrona & Troutman, 1986) directly linked infant temperament to postpartum depression. Fifty-five married women were assessed during pregnancy and at 3 months postpartum. The authors found that caring for a difficult infant gradually erodes a mother's feelings of competence as a parent and her overall sense of well-being. When a direct link between infant temperament and maternal depression was examined statistically, infant difficulty alone accounted for 30% of the variance in depression. Prolonged exposure to such an infant may make the mother feel ambivalent about the baby, resulting in guilt and self-dislike and her eventual withdrawal (as we described in Chapter 4). The authors concluded that the temperamentally difficult infant may disrupt several aspects of a woman's life, as Barbara describes:

> When the baby started throwing up, I felt terrible. I wouldn't go anyplace with her because I didn't want people to see her screaming. I wanted to be the perfect mother. . . . My mother-in-law said, "You've got to relax. She's picking up on your cues."
>
> The baby had a difficult temperament. Even now, she's very stubborn and strong willed. The control issue is big for me. I'm a perfectionist and always have been. I don't want the baby to experiment with food, even though I know it's normal. I don't want her to do it.
>
> I wanted this baby so bad. When she came, I hated her. I thought of throwing her out the window. I just wanted her to die. I spanked her when she was 3 or 4 weeks old, and I'm still dealing with the guilt of it. . . . I'd yell at her, right in her face, "I hate you. I wish you would die."

In a study of 43 mothers of 13-month-olds (Levitt et al., 1986), mothers with difficult infants were more likely to be depressed and to report less satisfactory relationships with their husbands than were mothers of easy infants. Mothers' perceptions of their infants as being difficult were related to both depressive symptoms and diagnoses of depression in a study of 115 women (Whiffen, 1988). In a more recent study, depressed women were more likely to describe their infants as difficult to care for at 2 months postpartum and to indicate that they felt overwhelmed by child care than were their nondepressed counterparts (Campbell et al., 1992). Mothers who perceived their infants as difficult tended to have more stressful reactions to negative events overall (Donovan & Leavitt, 1989), and the depressed women expressed fewer positive emotions with their infants, were less expressive or involved, and were less responsive or sensitive to their babies' needs than were the nondepressed women (Hoffman & Drotar, 1991).

Affonso and Arizmendi (1986) demonstrated that women at risk for postpartum depression were uncomfortable with their babies and become increasingly uncomfortable over time. They also found a positive correlation between depressive symptomatology and negative affect while with the baby. In another study infants of depressed mothers were receiving less responsive care at 2 months postpartum than were infants of nondepressed mothers (Campbell et al., 1992). If the downward cycle between mother and infant continues, it may lead to attachment difficulties, child maltreatment, or failure to thrive (Campbell et al., 1992; Klein, 1990). Even among mothers who are generally high functioning, depression can make them insensitive to their babies' needs. Debbie describes how her depression made her oblivious to her son's illness:

> I didn't care about anything. I didn't want to eat, I couldn't even get out of bed. I couldn't tell my son was jaundiced. My mother kept saying, "Your son is sick. You need to do something about your son," as she tried for the 10th time that day to get me out of bed. That's when I realized how bad the depression was and that I needed help. Everyone could tell the baby was sick but me. I didn't even notice it. I don't know what I would have done if my mother hadn't been here.

In another line of research, mothers' ratings of infant temperament were related to attachment, demonstrating the importance of mothers' perceptions of temperament. Mothers who described their infants as "difficult" at 4 months postpartum were less likely to have securely attached infants at 12 months. Further, mothers who perceived their infants as difficult tended to have more aversive reactions to an infant's crying (as measured by physiological criteria) and were more likely to use punitive child-rearing techniques as indicated in their attitudes toward spanking, comforting, and use of baby-sitters (Frodi, Bridges, & Shonk, 1989). Interestingly, in one study comparing depressed and nondepressed women, the depressed women had more overall negative perceptions of caring for their infants but did not perceive them as temperamentally difficult. Rather they tended to blame themselves for their infants' behaviors, despite the fact that the infants were in reality more difficult as determined by independent raters (Whiffen & Gotlib, 1989). The mothers' depression was related to the infants' negative behaviors, which was likely to exacerbate the mothers' negative mood.

Yet life with a difficult infant is not hopeless. Mothers can influence the amount of crying of even difficult babies. When mothers in one study consistently responded to and tried to comfort their crying babies at 3 months (Crockenberg & McCluskey, 1986), the babies (including those with difficult temperaments) cried less at 12 months during separation and were more securely attached.[1] Social support for mothers in the postpartum period is essential for enabling mothers to respond sensitively to their infants and is one of the best predictors of secure attachment at 12 months (Crockenberg, 1981). Without this support infants with difficult temperaments may become insecurely attached to their mothers (Goldsmith, Bradshaw, & Rieser-Danner, 1986), which can create problems for both mother and baby. For example, failure-to-thrive infants are more likely to be those with difficult temperaments (Singer, Song, Hill, & Jaffe, 1990), and hyperirritable, drug-addicted infants may be at greater risk for abuse by their mothers (Kantor, 1978).

Mothers who have infants with difficult temperaments may feel completely out of control, as Elizabeth describes:

> I felt completely out of control when he cried from 5 p.m. to 10 p.m. nightly with colic. A couple of times I shook him, and one time I hit him on the back. That was the most I did. I was completely desperate.

They also may blame themselves for their babies' behavior (Chalmers & Chalmers, 1986), as Melissa describes:

> I was convinced that my depression had damaged my child. He's a gloomy child. I thought I had done this. It took a long time for our pediatrician to convince me that that's his personality. It didn't occur to me that my second child is not like this and that he lived with me while I was depressed. I felt guilty about that for a long time.

The above discussion examined the relationship between babies who are essentially well but have difficult temperaments. The comments of the mothers we interviewed demonstrated the importance of both maternal and child characteristics in creating healthy relationships. In some cases the mothers interpreted their babies' behaviors as indicators that they had "failed" as mothers. When the mothers felt that they were not successful or out of control, they often felt more depressed and sometimes had negative feelings about their babies. When the mothers began to understand why their babies acted the way they did, it gave them a more realistic perspective on how much of their babies' behaviors they could control. They also felt more competent and less depressed. In the next section we describe the psychological reactions of women whose babies are ill.

AT-RISK INFANTS: THE EFFECTS ON MOTHERS OF INFANT PREMATURITY, ILLNESS, AND DISABILITY

> My first child was premature. He was born at 35 weeks with severe hyaline membrane disease. . . . He was in the hospital for 5 months; in the NICU for 4 months and in intermediate care for 1 month. . . . The depression started around the time he was 3 or 4 weeks old. . . . Up until that time, everything had been so urgent. He had had a couple of arrests. It was overwhelming. Suddenly my son was doing better. Why was I feeling so bad? I had difficulties going to sleep. I was up several times during the night. It was difficult to wake up in the morning. I didn't want to do anything during the day except sleep and call the NICU to check in. I started not to eat well. I felt an impending sense of doom. The depression lasted about a month.
>
> About a month after he came home, I felt physically depressed, same as in the initial postpartum period. I brought home a very

sick baby. I think it was a delayed reaction, reliving the early part [Patricia].

As we described in Chapter 2, postpartum depression is something of a paradox: Women get depressed at a time when everyone expects them to be ecstatic. The underlying assumption is that women have something to be happy about—namely, a healthy baby (Blumberg, 1980). However, women whose babies are not healthy, either because of prematurity, illness, or handicap, are often not diagnosed as having postpartum depression because there is an obvious source of their feelings of depression, concern, or sorrow. In this section we discuss some of the psychological implications for mothers of having an at-risk infant.[2] We particularly focus on reactions within the postpartum period, although we recognize that these reactions might be longer lasting. Similarly we focus on mothers' reactions, although we also recognize that fathers experience many of these same emotions.

The birth of an at-risk infant precipitates a psychological crisis. Women who give birth to an at-risk infant must face the reality of an infant who may be sickly or fragile when they themselves are psychologically and physically depleted. They may experience guilt for an early delivery, or anxiety regarding the viability and morbidity of their infants (Blumberg, 1980; Clark, 1979a, 1979b; Macey et al., 1987). The babies also may be born following a difficult pregnancy and/or delivery. Some of the aspects associated with medical care of a premature or sick newborn may contribute to the mother's grief and depression. Jan, who had a very difficult pregnancy and delivery, describes her feelings after the birth of her daughter. Her daughter was delivered 6 weeks premature, via emergency cesarean section, after Jan developed eclampsia:

> They took her away right after delivery. I never got to hold her, after all that [the difficult pregnancy and delivery]. They brought her back, but my arms were tied to the delivery table. I wish they had released at least one arm. It was really hard. . . . Leaving the hospital without the baby was really bad. I left early because I didn't want to leave at 11 a.m. with all the other moms and babies. . . . I shouldn't complain because she only had a few preemie problems. Others in the nursery were so sick. But it was very stressful. It was awful to see them putting the feeding tube down her throat, hearing her gagging and crying. It makes me cry now just to think about it.

In some cases, especially with babies who are very sick, mothers and fathers may experience anticipatory grieving and may begin to mourn the loss of their infants. In this process they may distance themselves from their babies in order to prepare themselves for their babies' eventual death. This process of mourning is interrupted, and parents have to readjust when the babies recover (Naylor, 1982). Patty, a pediatric nurse, describes her anticipatory grief reactions while her son was still in the hospital:

Friends or acquaintances would say that I was making more of a problem than it really was, that I was driving myself crazy, that I shouldn't anticipate things like the next crisis. It would be difficult when people gave me gifts. *I didn't know if I was going to take this kid home!* I didn't know if [the gift] would be around to remind me or if I would have to tearfully return it. That always put me into a depression.

The range of illnesses or problems of at-risk infants varies from very low birthweight (< 1,500 g) or premature infants, to infants who might have some minor complications. Some babies are hospitalized for only a few days, while others may be in intensive care for several weeks or months (Blumberg, 1980). Disabilities also vary considerably in their impairment of a child's functioning and the amount of extra stress that they place on the family. Even relatively minor problems that lead to mothers being separated from their babies can cause considerable emotional pain.

With the birth of a disabled baby, many mothers generally mourn the loss of their idealized or expected normal baby (Affleck et al., 1989; Naylor, 1982) and may be ashamed because they did not produce a "whole" child. Similarly they may feel that they did something to cause the problem or that they are being punished for something they did (Clark, 1979a, 1979b). Often women will search their memories, sometimes in vain, trying to recall the medications they took or the illnesses, however slight, that might account for the child's disability.

Mothers also may respond with a grief reaction. During the initial grieving stages, they proceed through the *disorganization and disequilibrium stage,* which includes shock, denial, anger, and sadness. The grief may continue as they think of all the things their child will not be able to do, and their expectations for the child continue to die (Panuthos & Romeo, 1984). As mothers resolve their initial grief, they come into the *coping and reorganization stage*. During this stage, mothers search for normal aspects of their infants that they can relate to, start becoming attached to their infants, and mobilize long-term medical attention on their babies' behalf (Clark, 1979b).

Most of the above-cited literature describes women's responses in terms of *grief reactions*, which include but are not limited to depression. Researchers also have examined the direct relationship between neonatal illness and maternal depression. Blumberg (1980) hypothesized that the greater the degree of neonatal risk, the more depressed the mothers would be. She collected data from 100 postpartum women whose infants had a variety of neonatal conditions. Risk was coded on a 5-point scale (*none* to *highest*). Blumberg's results revealed that neonatal risk was significantly correlated with depression (the higher the risk, the higher the depression), and infant risk alone accounted for a significant amount of depression. Similarly, mothers with babies who were most at risk had higher levels of anxiety and more negative perceptions of their newborns than did mothers whose babies were not at risk. This sample was ethnically and demographically diverse, indicating that the effects of neonatal risk were independent of other characteristics within the sample. Similarly, O'Hara et al. (O'Hara, 1986; O'Hara et al., 1984) found that stress associated with child care, such as when the baby had health problems, was related to increased postpartum depressive symptomatology. Jan experienced both anxiety and depression after the birth of her premature infant. Her symptoms started in the hospital and accelerated after she brought her daughter home:

> The panic attacks quieted down a little after I left the hospital without my daughter. They started getting really bad after I brought her home. Part of it was having a preemie at home. . . . When you have a preemie, you're up every 2 hours. It was scary to see her, to see how small she was. . . . I was afraid to be in the same room with my daughter. It was a big demand, feeding every 2 hours. That went on all day and night. When she was 6 months old, she only weighed 10 lbs. It was 15 months before she slept through the night. People would say I should let her cry, but I couldn't because of the anxiety. Her crying caused me severe anxiety. Even now, it gives me goose bumps to think about it.

Both Jan's and Patricia's stories (cited earlier) highlight that depression can take place at many different times throughout an infant's illness. Mothers may be particularly at risk immediately following their deliveries, after any medical crisis, when the mother must leave the hospital without the baby, when the baby is about to be discharged, or after the baby is home. A mother's risk of depression is further increased if the baby is transferred to another hospital, particularly if the hospital is in another city. If mothers follow their babies to these other hospitals, they may be cut off from their normal support systems, including their partners.

Degree of illness is one important factor related to depression. Another factor is the characteristics of at-risk babies themselves. Not only do mothers need to resolve their grief, but also the babies themselves bring unique difficulties to the mother-infant relationship. At-risk babies often act differently from well babies, and this can make their parents confused about how to interpret their babies' signals (Macey et al., 1987). For example, premature babies can be very unpredictable in their daily patterns, and this can be taxing for parents (Boukydis, Lester, & Hoffman, 1987). They also may be overly sensitive to stimulation and not as responsive as well babies. Because these babies may not be as responsive as "normal" babies, mothers may overstimulate them and so cause the infants to withdraw even further. The mothers may respond to this withdrawal by either increasing the amount of stimulation or withdrawing from the baby, thus creating a vicious cycle (Jarvis, Myers, & Creasey, 1989). This problem of dysfunctional interactions may have started in the hospital because the mother was limited in the amount of contact she could have. Some babies are so very ill or sensitive that mother-infant contact is greatly curtailed. These types of problems often result in interactions between mother and baby that are not reinforcing and that can make mothers feel helpless, thus furthering the helpless feeling that may have begun in the hospital (Capuzzi, 1989).

Such maladaptive interactions are understandable, in light of the fragility of the infants. Nevertheless they can have long-term effects. For example, mothers of preterm infants show less confidence in their ability to parent than do mothers of full-term infants, particularly if they have been denied contact with their babies (Campos et al., 1983). In addition, mothers of preterm infants tend to hold their babies less, make less eye contact, or smile less often than do mothers of fullterms (Parke & Tinsley, 1987). When preterm infants are 1-4 months old, their mothers are more active and intrusive in their interactional style. But problems in interactions might be related to degree of illness of the premature baby, not prematurity per se. Mothers also may feel that they must "ask permission" from experts (doctors and nurses) before they care for their babies and are therefore less likely to interact confidently once the baby is released from the hospital.

In one study (Jarvis et al., 1989) the authors compared three groups of prematures: those with no medical complications, those who were moderately ill (respiratory distress syndrome), and those who were very ill (bronchopulmonary dysplasia) at 4 and 8 months of age. As predicted, degree of illness did influence the mother-infant interaction at both time points. Mothers of the sickest infants were less sensitive to their infants' cues, did not respond well to their infants' distress, and did not foster socioemotional growth, compared with mothers in the other two groups. Further, mothers of the sickest infants became less responsive to their infants between 4 and 8 months, perhaps reflecting their increasing withdrawal from the infant (possibly because of anticipatory grieving), whereas mothers of the moderately ill infants actually became more sensitive in their responses over this same time period.

Differences in mother-infant interaction due to the infant's illness also were found with a group of nonpremature infants (Fischer-Fay, Goldberg, Simmons, & Levison, 1988). In this study 15-month-old infants with cystic fibrosis (CF) were compared with healthy infants of the same age. The results revealed no differences in attachment patterns for infants with CF and healthy infants. Within the group of CF infants, however, those with the lowest weights were significantly more likely to have insecure attachments to their mothers. In another study (Bendersky & Lewis, 1986) birth order interacted with degree of prematurity and illness. As predicted, primiparous women were more attentive to the needs of their high-risk infants than were mothers whose high-risk infants were laterborn. The results of this study most likely reflect the increased burdens of having to care both for an older healthy child (or children) and a laterborn high-risk infant.

The results of these studies and the comments of the mothers we interviewed indicate that an at-risk infant can be taxing for parents and also can be related to maternal depression. In some cases women may resent the extra burdens that their infants place on the family. They also may feel guilty for these feelings and withdraw from others. It is during this phase that social support for mothers is crucial. In the next section we review research that specifically has addressed the issue of social support for mothers of at-risk infants.

Social Support for Mothers of At-Risk Infants

I found it difficult to speak with my husband and family about being depressed and about my constant concern and worry. They kept trying to be positive, saying what they would do with him when he got well. I don't know if my medical knowledge made it worse. I knew how serious it was. It made me more depressed when my family was upbeat and tried to deny how serious it was. I had to deal with their denial, and I felt they were heaping expectations on me.

I got lots of support from a couple we're friends with. She's a NICU nurse. They would offer to sit at the hospital for us so we could go out. They also made meals for us. They were people who understood the medical issues. They didn't say everything would be OK. They realized it could be fatal [Patricia].

Social support can mediate many of the negative effects of having an at-risk infant. As we described in Chapter 4, social support can take many forms, including information, practical assistance, and emotional support. Patricia indicated (see above quotation) that some types of support that people offered were more effective than others. As we indicated in the previous chapter, assistance is only true support when mothers *perceive* it that way.

The results of two recent studies indicate that social support can positively affect attachment between mothers and at-risk infants. In the first study, mothers of handicapped infants initially showed fewer attachment behaviors at 1 month postpartum than did the comparison group of mothers of nonhandicapped babies, regardless of the length of hospital stay (Capuzzi, 1989). By 6 and 12 months, however, these differences had disappeared. Social support for the mother reduced the stress of having a handicapped child and facilitated attachment. On the basis of her findings, the author suggested that attachment is a dynamic process that develops over time. Although mothers of handicapped infants may have a more difficult time developing this attachment, they can adapt and develop it. Similar results were found in a study of 52 high-risk premature infants (Crnic, Greenberg, & Slough, 1986).

Social support also has been helpful in facilitating attachment and infant development in babies identified as being at-risk because of environmental factors such as maternal depression and poverty (Lyons-Ruth, Connell, Grunebaum, & Botein, 1990). In this study 31 depressed mothers were given weekly home-visiting services. They were compared with depressed mothers of similar low socioeconomic status at 18 months. The home-visiting services provided information and emotional support and overcame the effects of maternal depression for the infants. Those who received these services had infants with scores an average of 10 points higher on the Bayley Scales (a measure of infant development and intelligence) and were twice as likely to be classified as securely attached. They did not report whether the mothers who received services were less depressed, however.

Another study (Affleck et al., 1989) indicates that formal social support for mothers of high-risk babies is effective only if the mothers perceive a need for support. When the mothers needed support, the program (consisting of support and information from in-home nurse consultants) improved mothers' sense of perceived control, competence, and responsiveness. The program had a negative effect on mothers who had a low need for support, by actually making them feel less competent and more anxious.

In summary, both mothers and at-risk babies bring special challenges to the mother-infant relationship. Mothers may be in the process of grieving when they are forced to deal with babies who are different from what they expected and may be difficult to handle. In spite of these difficulties, attachment can develop between mother and baby, especially if the mother is given adequate support (and she perceives it as support). Nurses can do much to facilitate these types of positive reactions. Helping mothers feel competent in caring for their at-risk babies is vital for reducing risk for postpartum depression and for helping mothers become attached to their babies.

SUGGESTIONS FOR NURSES

The nursing literature offers many specific suggestions on how to help mothers of difficult or at-risk babies. We have summarized these suggestions below and have added some of our own. The first set deals with home-based interventions, such as those that visiting nurses might initiate. The second set of suggestions is for maternity or NICU nurses. All of these suggestions, however, can be applied by nurses in either situation or possibly by those who work in obstetricians' or pediatricians' offices, although their contact is likely to be more limited.

The focus of this chapter has been on the mother-infant relationship and behaviors that promote effective interactions. Therefore we emphasize this area, while recognizing that your intervention may include other issues, such as working with mothers to provide for the physical needs of their babies. Further, although we have limited our discussion in this chapter to mothers whose infants might be temperamentally difficult or ill, these suggestions can apply to any mother who is having difficulties with her baby (Klein, 1990).

Education for Mothers

Providing education for mothers is an important step for promoting attachment and for helping mothers feel more competent. This education can provide support by acknowledging that the mothers have a challenging job and by recognizing the special demands their babies create. We have directed these comments toward the behaviors of mothers because mothers are the most changeable component of the mother-infant dyad. Although it might be possible to make small changes in the infant's behaviors, these require time (in some cases, a year or more). A woman dealing with a difficult or at-risk infant needs answers right away and is not comforted by promises that the baby will grow out of it.[3]

The more that mothers know about their babies' capabilities, the more competent they will feel and the better equipped they will be to meet their babies' needs. Education also can create more realistic expectations about what their babies are capable of. Klein (1990) recommended that nurses provide education with the following components:

Teaching mothers the meaning of a child's behavior. This is especially important for mothers of difficult infants who may interpret their babies' behaviors as "manipulating" or rejecting them
or as being their fault. It is important to teach mothers about
temperament differences and to provide support for them, because some of the people they know may be telling the mothers
that the babies' behaviors are their fault. In addition, it is
important to teach mothers how to respond effectively to their
babies so that they are not overstimulating them, thereby creating more positive interactions between them.

Colic is a common physiological problem that affects temperament and can make even easy infants appear difficult. Explaining to mothers the physiological causes of colic (e.g., an immature
gastrointestinal system) can eliminate the tendency of mothers
to blame themselves and may make them better able to cope.
Mothers who blame themselves for their babies' colic may
withdraw from the infant and other people who could provide
them with support and respite.

Every effort should be made to eliminate any environmental
elements that may be aggravating the colic. The baby should be
tested for milk allergies or other conditions that might be contributing to the problem. Further, mothers who use formula
may need to switch brands or type, and mothers who breast-
feed should be counseled about eliminating certain foods from
their diets that may be contributing to the problem (e.g., cucum-
bers, brussels sprouts, chocolate, caffeine, or milk products). If
breast-feeding difficulties arise, the mother should be given
lactation instruction or be referred to a group that provides
lactation support (such as La Leche League).

Teaching mothers nurturing behaviors. This is especially important
for mothers who may not have received this type of nurturance as
children or for women who have had limited experience with
babies. This type of teaching could include the modeling of touch-
ing, cuddling, stroking, making eye contact with, smiling at, and
talking to the baby. The teaching also could include pointing out
the child's positive responses to the mother's behaviors such as
reaching, cooing, smiling, or making eye contact.

Teaching coping skills. For any intervention to be effective, parents must learn how to deal with the extra stress associated with

taking care of a high-needs baby. One key coping skill is learning how to manage and alleviate stress in ways that involve solving the problem and not taking it out on the family. Another coping strategy is learning how to get assistance. This might involve learning how to locate sources of help, including agencies that can assist with food, housing, family planning, medical care, emotional support, or marital counseling. Examples of these types of resources are WIC, local health departments or social service agencies, the Red Cross, Salvation Army, Catholic Charities, and Jewish Family and Children's Services. Also helpful are parent-stress hot lines and parent support and education groups. (See the Appendix for other suggestions for finding community support.)

Helping Mothers Resolve Their Grief

The next set of suggestions pertains to mothers of premature, ill, or disabled infants. Clark (1979a, 1979b) offered several specific suggestions for nurses who work with mothers of at-risk babies, especially maternity and NICU nurses. According to Clark, nurses have two main goals: helping mothers resolve their grief and facilitating mother-infant attachment.

First, she suggested that nurses should help mothers air their feelings about having an at-risk infant. Mothers may have many strong feelings about what has happened, including anger, guilt, grief, or fear. They must feel free to express these feelings, because this is the first step in accepting what has happened (Panuthos & Romeo, 1984). To help mothers cope, nurses should help mothers deal with the realities of their situations and what it will be like to take this baby home.

Mothers also may feel helpless while their babies are in the hospital. To counteract this helplessness, nurses should try to involve mothers in the caregiving of their babies. For example, mothers and fathers should be given as much access to their babies as is possible, even if it is only to sit beside the isolette. Involve mothers in feeding and bathing their babies. Provide a place where mothers can nurse. If the baby is too ill to nurse, encourage breast-feeding mothers to pump their breast milk and to bring it to the hospital. Providing electric breast pumps and places to store milk, and teaching mothers to express their milk are two ways to involve the participation of the mothers and to increase their confidence. Another way to involve the mothers' participation is to explain tests and procedures to them, to offer them information, and to elicit their questions. Parents might feel very dependent during this time of grief and disorganization. This dependence is appropriate for the time being, but your eventual goal is to move them toward independence and confidence in caregiving. Approaching them with warmth and acceptance and letting them know that their feelings are not unnatural will help them deal with their grief and move on.

The next step is to facilitate attachment between mother and infant. Some of this process will occur as mothers become involved in the care of their infants. Nurses can act as role models for mothers about how to handle their babies. According to Clark, mothers will watch nurses very closely to see whether they show any signs of rejecting the babies. This is especially the case with disabled infants. Therefore the nurse is in a good position to model acceptance of the baby for the mother. At the same time a balance has to be struck so that the nurse is not perceived as the only competent "mother" and the mother's feelings of self-efficacy are enhanced.

Later, the nurse can help the mother learn about any special care needs that the baby has. The nurse needs to provide the mother with opportunities for success so that she gains a sense of confidence. In addition, putting her in contact with other mothers whose babies have been ill can be very helpful after she leaves the hospital. Before the baby leaves the hospital, the mother should know where to find support and information within her community so that she can have ongoing assistance. Obtaining a referral to a visiting nurse association may be very helpful as well.

In the next chapter we examine how postpartum illness can be the result of many factors all at once.

NOTES

1. *Attachment* refers to the emotional bond between the infant and caregiver (usually the mother). Mother-infant attachments typically are characterized as being either *secure* or *insecure*. When infants are securely attached, they will use

their mothers as safe bases from which to explore the environment. The secure attachment also forms the basis for psychological development later in life (Santrock & Yussen, 1992). Behaviors that indicate an insecure attachment include avoiding the mother (avoidant type; averting gaze, ignoring her, failing to seek proximity) or resisting her (ambivalent type; clinging while pushing away).

Security of attachment is generally determined by using the *strange situation* paradigm (Ainsworth, 1979), during which the baby is observed alone in an unfamiliar room, interacting with the mother alone, with the mother and a stranger, and with the stranger alone. Types of behaviors observed are the baby's exploratory behaviors and proximity seeking, her or his reactions to the stranger, reactions to being left alone, and behaviors on being reunited with the mother. Although some have raised questions about this paradigm and the classification of infants (see Campos et al., 1983), it nevertheless is used as an outcome measure in many studies.

2. In this section we use the term *at-risk* as a general term to describe infants at risk for difficulties in the mother-infant relationship because of prematurity, neonatal illness, or disability. Although we originally had planned to separate our discussions of these three conditions, they often are combined in research studies. Therefore we used *at-risk* as a term to describe all three conditions, while recognizing that this term is far from ideal.

3. Readers interested in the effects of maternal depression on infants are referred to two excellent reviews on the topic by Tronick and Field (1986) and Field (1992).

The Multiple Causes of Postpartum Illness: One Woman's Story

Postpartum illness is a complex phenomenon that may a have single cause or multiple causes. In the last four chapters we have described the most frequently cited factors related to postpartum illness. Yet by separating these causes, we might have made it difficult to conceptualize how multiple factors can interact within one person. In this chapter we bring all the threads together by describing one woman's experience in detail. The focus of this chapter is on the illness itself to give the reader insight into how a women might subjectively experience postpartum illness. Jenny's account is juxtaposed with the account of her physicians and other caregivers.

Jenny's story offers a unique glimpse into postpartum illness and nicely illustrates its multicausal nature. Typical studies of postpartum illness are based on retrospective accounts. What makes Jenny's story unique is that she kept a journal before her baby was born, after the birth, and during her hospitalization for postpartum psychosis. Jenny's journal provides detailed qualitative information that she wrote while going through her illness. She has shared her diary with us, as well as the medical records from the state hospital, with the hope that they will help other women suffering from postpartum depression and psychosis.

BACKGROUND

Jenny relates her illness to a number of different factors. Jenny feels that she was vulnerable to postpartum illness because of her health history and her lifelong struggle with severe allergies. (Some researchers and physicians have noted a relationship between allergies and mental illness as well; Adler, 1991b; Mandel & Scanlon, 1979). In addition to her health history, she experienced a series of stressors in both the pre- and postpartum periods, which are described below.

Jenny was 20 years old when she had her daughter. Her marriage and the birth of her daughter within less than a year constituted two major life changes within a relatively short span of time. Nevertheless she was happy with her new life and joyfully celebrated the birth of her first child. She also was buffered from the potential negative effects of these stressors by a large and supportive family, a close relationship with her parents, and a strong religious faith:

> [My baby] was born exactly 76 hours ago. December 1, 1988, at 10:44 p.m. This will be a landmark day in my life. I was so overjoyed and emotionally ready for her to be here, and now she's here. . . . [My husband], Mom, Dad, and [two friends] were all there. It was an awesome moment.

As thrilled as she was with the birth of her daughter, her birth experience was stressful. Jenny does not feel that it was the sole or even main cause of her illness (as it was for some of the women described in Chapter 3). Rather it was the first link in a chain of events that led to her illness.

THE BIRTH EXPERIENCE

Jenny was very involved in the care that she received during her pregnancy. Before the baby was born, she carefully prepared herself for labor and delivery, read extensively, exercised, and did yoga. Four weeks before her due date, she read two books on the Bradley method of natural childbirth. Although she had always wanted to have natural childbirth, these were the first books she had read that articulated what she wanted. Unfortunately the hospital where she was to deliver specialized in high-risk patients and tended to intervene frequently, even in routine births: The hospital's rate of cesarean births was an alarming 50%. Because it was so close to her due date, she had no choice but to proceed with her doctor and the hospital. Even after making the decision to proceed, she knew that it would be difficult to have a natural delivery in that setting:

> My alarm grew as the week progressed. [My husband] and I went on a tour of [the hospital] and I freaked out. I had done everything backwards. I chose my doctor then the hospital, then 3 weeks before giving birth, I discovered the method I wanted to use. Not exactly ideal. According to Bradley, you choose the facility, then the doctor, and you know the method before you get pregnant. Anyway, the past 4 weeks have been hell as I've tried to convince [my husband], my doctor, my mom, and mostly myself that this was the method I wanted to use. At one point, I seriously considered changing doctor/hospital but we recognized that most doctors won't take on a patient this late in the game.
>
> Knowing I'd have a fight on my hands, I read the Bradley method three times to fully acquaint myself with the techniques—(all relaxation, deep breathing, concentration) and all the arguments for not having "procedures" done at the hospital, to me or the baby.

During her lengthy labor (over 24 hours), one of the more negative aspects was the way she was treated by the hospital staff. At one point she was alone in a hospital room on a table. She had only a sheet over her, and she was very cold. An intern who was apparently inexperienced came in and gave her a rough and lengthy examination. Another doctor examined her, and then the intern and the other doctor discussed Jenny's progress with each other in front of her:

> Then I began having a hard contraction. She [the second doctor] put her hands on my abdomen and instructed the intern to do likewise. They both were pushing and poking. I about lost control. I realized that he was the teachee and she was the teacher and I

was the guinea pig. When my contraction was over, I said, "Don't ever touch me while I'm having a contraction again."

At this point she asked to see her husband, who had been outside the room talking to her doctor on the telephone:

> When I saw him [her husband], I almost started to cry. I had asked three nurses for a blanket because I was frozen. I was cold, hurting, and those dumb doctors had been using my laboring body to teach each other what a contraction should feel like.

At this point Jenny and her husband were given the option of going home, walking, or being admitted to a labor room. She could not be admitted to the birthing room, as she requested, because she was only 2-3 cm dilated. They decided to go home. The Bradley method states that solitude, quiet, physical comfort, and physical relaxation are essential for the laboring woman. During the hours at the hospital, none of these were available. She labored at home for the next few hours and started to make progress. She arrived at the hospital again, hoping to go directly to the birthing room after being checked at her doctor's office:

> When we arrived at the hospital, I was cold, tense, and nervous that I would get a lot of crap from the hospital staff. I sat in a wheelchair during *nine* contractions. As usual they had miscommunicated the doctor's request for me. One nurse said I had to go to triage to "get checked." Another said I couldn't drink anything when she saw me take a sip of Vernors pop. Another said the birthing room wasn't prepped. (We had called 1/2 hour before from the clinic to tell them we were on our way.) No time to prep? Bull! I sat in that wheelchair getting madder and madder. Finally I asked the admitting nurse if I could go labor in a labor bed until the room was ready because I was having a hard time controlling my contractions. She called the birthing room to ask. They said, "No, we're just about done." I had *two* more contractions while they finished. I was almost crying by now. I kept thinking of how wonderful I had felt at home, the contractions didn't even hurt while I was in the shower with the hot air [sic] beating on my back.

She sat in a wheelchair in the lobby of the hospital for 30 minutes while in active labor. Once she got into the birthing room, she continued to have trouble with the hospital staff over the issue of continuous fetal monitoring. Prior to coming back to the hospital, her doctor had agreed to intermittent fetal monitoring (10 minutes every hour), but the nurses kept insisting that she have continuous fetal monitoring. At one point they even threatened to make her leave if she did not comply. When she was 5 cm dilated, her doctor ruptured her membranes. Three hours later her daughter was born. In spite of the difficulties, it was a joyous occasion.

THE POSTPARTUM PERIOD

Approximately 8 weeks after her daughter was born, Jenny and her husband moved to another state. This move pulled Jenny away from her support network, including her close-knit family. During this time her husband's back went out, adding to the stress of their move, as he was unable to help with either child care or the move. Nevertheless Jenny was happy in her new role and enjoyed their new home:

> It's so wonderful to be a mother. I've dreamed and planned to be one all my life. She [her daughter] is everything to me, besides [my husband], and I would die for her. She's pretty and personable and I'm flattered that she wants to be with me most. It makes me feel good to see that satisfied look on her little face when she's done eating and I love to think that her little body is receiving nourishment and growth from my body.

Within approximately 6 weeks of their move to another state, Jenny developed postpartum psychosis. During the weeks prior to her psychosis, she had read a book about allergies which listed a number of food and environmental allergens. This book recommended a 5-day fast as a way of locating allergy-producing substances (Mandel & Scanlon, 1979). Having suffered from allergies all her life, she took this very seriously. She started to fast, even though she was nursing, in an attempt to locate the foods and substances that caused allergic reactions. She also was getting fewer and fewer hours of sleep each night, insisting she could handle everything. As the days passed, she became increasingly manic. In this state she took everything to its extreme, including trying to purify her body and her household environment by getting rid of all plastic and by turning off her heat because there was a natural gas leak in her home. Here is her retrospective description of what happened to her. She wrote this account shortly after she was released from the psychiatric hospital:

> It started slowly, then built to a peak. I became paranoid about being clean, purity, being perfect. I wanted to be a savior: save the town, the ward, the state, everyone. I wanted the millennium to start. I wanted to go to the temple to see Christ face to face. I wanted to live the word of wisdom perfectly. I cut out sugar, chocolate, meat, and ate only whole organic foods. I fasted. [My baby] looked hungry when my mom arrived. I kept freaking out, thinking [my husband] was going to die, someone was going to kill me, steal [my baby], etc. . . . It was hell!
>
> I sang hymns all the time to ward off evil thoughts and spirits. I ran to Main Street, staying in the light, casting Satan out of [town], took my clothes off to my garments,[1] sat down in the lotus position looking at the sun, and waited. A police woman came up and tried to talk to me. She called [my husband]. He came and tried to get me to come home. They threw me in the ambulance and I came to. I put on my clothes, declared I was fine, and did my banking. [My husband] flipped out. He called the bishop and my parents. I asked my mom to come down.

Her parents and husband took her to the hospital where she had delivered, but she refused to check herself in. From there she went to the state hospital for 9 days in her parents' state, then a private hospital for 9 days, then back to the state hospital for 6 days, and finally back to the private hospital for 2 weeks. After her release she convalesced at her parents' home for 1 month before returning home with her husband.

THE HOSPITAL DIARY

The next section of Jenny's story is taken from the diary she kept while in the state and private mental hospitals (the first time at each one). She wrote this account while she was hospitalized for postpartum psychosis. Much of the journal is dedicated to trying to make sense of what had happened to her. The following are excerpts from her diary.

March 29, 1989 This is going to be the most important journal I've ever kept. I'm in a mental hospital. [name of state hospital] On Friday, I'm moving to a new hospital. [name of private hospital]. I'm confused though. Talking helps. I'm hoping this journal will help. I asked mom to bring it to me. Everyone here is very nice. They are all trying to help me get better.

March 30, 1989, 7:19 a.m. I woke up this morning and my breasts were aching (forced weaning). I asked the nurse for some Tylenol. She brought me some and I feel better. I exercised, prayed, watched the news, ate a banana that Mom gave me yesterday (day before yesterday), and I feel good. . . . I cried this morning because I miss [my baby]. I want to nurse her so bad but I've accepted that I won't be able to ever again—that hurts. I loved to think that it was my body that helped to make her grow. What a lift! But I can deal with it. I miss her smilin' face.

7:43 a.m. I've been thinking of an analogy to what has happened. It goes like this. Imagine yourself getting kicked in the head. But there is no tissue damage, no blood, no bruise, only your brain has been hurt. The hurt is very bad and you try to make it better but don't know what to do. You scream and cry and try to hurt yourself. You act totally irrational. As time goes by, the hurt starts to heal, somehow. The cells repair themselves (analogy), the tissue rebuilds, all that is really needed is some time, rest, good food, a listening ear, and a notebook with a pen. The memory comes back and with it dark images, so evil, and bad that you cry, but also light, God, hope, love and peace. These images fight each other for space in your conscious. As time goes by, the light is the one that prevails and sanity or at least peace is restored. The dark images return sometimes to scare and frighten but eventually the light prevails and everything is OK. Now, I just need time to understand why and sort things out. It hurts to think I went through so much. Sometimes I'm embarrassed by my behavior. I want to crawl under a rock. But I'm also relieved because so much that was unexplainable is now understood.

I'm still not myself. I have so many questions. And every time I ask one of the patients, they either look at me crazy or they give me their philosophy on life. The nurses try to answer my questions, but they are very busy and the doctors are great but they have even less time and many demands. It's OK, Mom said [private hospital] will be much better and they'll answer my questions and clear up any confusions. I can't wait to go. I just know it's *got* to be better than this place. I don't hate it here, but I can see that it's holding me back from getting better.

8:55 a.m. I can't help having the feeling that the nurses and everyone keep lying to me and there is some major plot against me. They tell me one thing, then do another. They told me the gynecologist would be here at 8:30. Well, it's long past. They don't understand that to me a minute is like an hour and a day is like a month. Even 5 minutes seems like a year. Time is relative I know, but I wish they would tell the truth. I'm so confused as it is. I wish they'd come soon. I don't want them to take any blood. I hope they don't. I really am afraid to go see these doctors. I don't know them and they are going to touch the most private parts of my body. I usually don't have a problem with this, but now I'm scared. It's weird how you can change so quickly. I still am confused. I want answers *NOW!!*

12:10 p.m. I finally saw the doctors at 9:30 a.m. It's so hard to *wait!* They were cool. Wanted to take some blood but I said "no." Wanted to do a pelvic, I said "no way." I'm feeling too vulnerable right now. I need some time before they do these things again. I still think I'm going to refuse drugs at any cost. I'm having a hard enough time getting control and I really think what I need is some sleep.

I would say 95% of this problem is physical. The doctors and everyone keep talking about "chemical" but I think sleep deprivation is a real disease and I haven't had "good" sleep in *so long.* And the food changes that I imposed upon myself were a large part of this too so I understand why—at least some of the whys, but I still have quite a few to figure out. I have a lot of questions, but each second something new comes to me. The greatest thing is the way [my husband] and the family are supporting me. They are the greatest in the world. They have been visiting, bringing me food, talking on the phone and in person. They don't realize how much that helps. For 4 days, I was in isolation. I didn't know where I was, what was going on or where any of my family were, and I was scared to death. So scared, hurt, afraid, lonely, I wanted to die, that was *all* that I wanted.

About 10 times during the isolation, I thought OK, this is it, here I go, and then something would happen and I would be released for another few minutes, hours, seconds until the next death wish came. It peaked on Saturday night when I wanted to die for the last time. My tongue was lolling around in my head, I was dazed and confused. I hurt all over, my body was convulsing but all I wanted to do was die. The doctor was truly hurting my arm with the I.V. and instead of dying, I fell asleep. It was so depressing. When I woke up on Easter Sunday, I couldn't understand why I was alive. I didn't know what Christ wanted me to do. I had done everything I could to purify my life and body and he still didn't want to see me face to face.

[After receiving a blessing that night from her father, the death wishes stopped.] . . . Then I became suspicious of everyone. I thought they were trying to poison me with the food. I thought they were draculas taking my blood. I pulled out the I.V. and the catheter because I *knew* God wanted me to do it.

March 31, 1989, 8:00 a.m. Today has finally arrived! I get to leave this pit of despair. *Everyone* is so pathetic here. . . . I was *so* angry last night. I kept imagining doing terrible things. The thing is I'm a good person. I want to do what's right. I have a daughter who needs me, a husband who needs me, and I don't need to be in this shit-hole prison. So why the hell am I here?????? I didn't commit any crime and I practically have to ask permission to pee. They try to poison me with this shit they call food and surround me with so much smoke it's like a bar. I hate it *here*. . . . I keep seeing myself in [town name], singing hymns, and casting out Satan. The police-woman came up to me and asked me to get dressed. Poor lady. As I was sitting there in the full lotus position with my hands in the symbol of knowledge pose, all I can remember is this guy walking by and saying to her "This isn't exactly Mr. Rogers' neighborhood, is it?" And me, wanting to laugh but knowing I couldn't because it was too solemn a moment, and Satan would get my soul if I moved before [my husband] got there. Then he arrived and said, "Jenn, you've gotta come home," and I did, but I was *very* sick.

At this point she was transferred to the private mental hospital. The following are excerpts taken from her diary written at that time:

March 31, 5:00 p.m. I'm finally here. It's nice. I'm exhausted. The orientation helped. I have so many questions but mostly I want to rest. I feel nervous, tense, overwhelmed. I had an in-tense [sic] evaluation, a medical check-up, an evaluation with a shrink (he was nice, not Dr. S., but a good guy).

April "Fools" Day, 1989. Just met with Dr. S. He's an ass. Really. Wants me to take drugs. I just kept saying "nope." He can't force me unless I have another psychotic episode. I'm going to do everything I can to avoid that. But I *refuse* to fall into their mode of medicate, medicate, medicate. All I need is some sleep, some good food, and a chance to get my wits about me. . . . He kept tryin' to say I needed drugs. He doesn't know a damn thing about me except that I did some outrageous things out of the norm.

I'm not just going to roll with it folks. I'm going to fight them *every* step of the way and I'm going to question *everything*. Sorry if that's in-con-*VIEN*-ient, but it's the way it goes. I'm going to get along with everyone and get the hell out of here.

Later. . . . This place is awful. What I was just thinking is if it is such a great place and does so much good, why the hell has my roommate been here *six* times? . . . She is *so* doped up and screwed in the head by all the probing, searching to find out why, that I think she's on the verge of suicide. Well, she told me she was. Everyone here seems doped up, suicidal and depressed. I think this *all* could have been avoided *if* Mom and Dad had taken me home, put me to bed and let me sleep it off. But I was in a psychotic state when they showed up and I know they were scared by my behavior. So, like everyone else, take her to DRS. GOD. *They* will make everything better. Bullshit! All they did was scare the shit out of me and isolate me from my family.

This place is the same. They have buckets of pills, lots of analysis and isolation. *Most* of the people here need these things because they are suicidal. I am not suicidal. I'm just a tired Mom who was put in a situation [new hometown] that was hard to handle and freaked out. I had too too too much pressure. No sleep (for a month) and I changed my eating habits. Those things plus all the pressure of the move, my callings, [my husband's] calling, Bradley method of childbirth classes, fear of Satanism in [new town], pressure to be the best wife, best mother, best friend, best ward member, best sister, best daughter, best actress, best children's theater director, best temple-goer, cleanest house, cleanest healthiest body, cleanest healthiest well-behaved baby, best body, best reader, best student, best sister-in-law, best daughter-in-law, best gardener, best reader, most intelligent church-goer, best talker, best listener, best EVERYTHING, was *too* much. I need a vacation. That's what [hospital] is to me. I'm going to sleep, read, eat, and write—journal, letters, and I'm not going to listen to my doctor too much.

I'm very suspicious of a doctor who doesn't even know me coming in and telling me I "need" drugs to make me "feel good." Sorry, that just doesn't cut it. If he said "you have an infection, I want you to help it get better," I'd take them. But I *don't* believe in "feel good" drugs and dammit *nobody* is going to make me take them. I'm not going to become one of "these" zombies who walk around pretending everything is fine. I know that I have a problem. I want to know what caused it, what I can do to avoid it in the future, and how I can get better.

April 1st, 7:40 p.m. Well it's been a helluva day. I've been harassed by just about everybody to take the drugs (yes, including [my husband] and Mom). . . . [After a discussion with her doctor] he began pushing the drugs earnestly. He even tried to "bargain" with me. "I'll let you see your baby if you take the medicine." Nope. Those types of statements make me so curious to know *why* he feels the drugs are so important. I am *convinced* that the psycho-sis I experienced in [state name] was worst when I had no sleep, was eating little or fasting and when I was really tired. Nobody else seems to be. . . . I admit I have a problem. I want to get better and I want to know why but I *have* to do it *my* way. This is just like the birth. Hopefully, they'll understand.

THE PSYCHIATRIC EVALUATION

During the time this diary was written, the doctors at the mental hospitals were keeping their own records. The following are excerpts from these records that describe Jenny's illness from the medical perspective. The first entries were made at the time Jenny was discharged from the state hospital to the private hospital. Below are excerpts from the "combined psychiatric examination and summary note."

Mental Status:

This is a 21 year old, white female who appears to be her stated age. She is of moderate build. The patient is very agitated and disoriented. Her affect is blunted. Her mood went from hostile to tearful and scared. The patient denied being depressed but stated that she was very tired. The patient denied any suicidal or homicidal thoughts. She was preoccupied with religious grandiose delusions, stating "I was chosen by Jesus to fill a mission on this earth. I don't need a doctor. Jesus will heal me. I will fast until he comes to heal me." The patient is oriented to person and time. The patient seems to be confused regarding the events of the last four or five days. The patient's long-term memory appears to be intact. Her judgment and insight are poor.

Clinical Course and Treatment in the Hospital:

The patient was admitted on 3/23/89 from [other hospital] on a Medical Certificate. The patient was admitted with four-point restraints due to her being uncooperative to admission procedures. She was nonverbal and her behavior was unpredictable. The patient was put into seclusion. She was refusing meals and drank five, eight ounce glasses of water. On 3/24/89 the patient remained in seclusion. She was very agitated and delusional. She received 2.5 mg of Haldol and refused to talk to the doctor and refused to take a shower or use the bathroom. On 3/25/89, the patient continued to be hostile, refused to put clothes on, or to eat or drink. The patient voided on the floor, refusing to use the bathroom. Haldol was given to the patient. She received Benadryl 25 mg due to a dystonic reaction from Haldol. The patient continued to refuse fluids and was transferred to [other facility] to monitor input and output and dehydration. The patient had IV and Foley catheter. She was placed in four-point restraints due to her kicking the staff and not keeping her clothes on. On 3/26/89, the patient continued to refuse fluids or food. On 3/27/89, she was up and responding to verbal questioning. The patient cleaned herself up. While in the bathroom, the patient pulled out the IV and Foley. The patient began drinking fluids and her mother brought food from home. She began to eat the food brought from home well. The patient was transferred back to Receiving C. The patient became oriented and began to remember what had been happening in the last week. From 3/28/89 to 3/30/89, the patient continued to be cooperative, discussed stressors, and discussed mental illness. Arrangements were made to transfer the patient to [private hospital]. On 3/31/89, the patient was transferred to [private hospital] for continued hospitalization.

This next section is taken from the "psychosocial history." The informants were Jenny's husband and her parents. Jenny was not interviewed herself "due to her extreme psychosis."

According to the informants, the patient found her natural childbirth experience frustrating due to her unrealistic expectations. The method that the patient chose conflicted with the standard hospital fetal monitoring techniques. This created numerous conflicts for the patient throughout the labor and delivery. Consequently, the patient left the hospital twelve hours after the birth, with the baby. The family indicated that the patient and her child were released appropriately, even though the physician recommended that they stay an additional one or two more days. The patient and the child were released under the care of the patient's mother, who provided the patient with rest and helped in caring for the newborn.

This is the patient's first psychiatric hospitalization. The onset was sudden, with a direct connection to the recent birth of her daughter. According to the informants, throughout the delivery of the child, the patient was hostile and suspicious of physicians. The patient had opted for a particular type of natural childbirth, three weeks prior to the birth of the baby. She discussed this with her obstetrician, who did not prepare her for certain discrepancies between hospital policy and the method of natural childbirth. The informants report that, even after the birth, the patient sustained her hostile and angry feelings.

The informants report that the symptoms escalated when the patient and her husband moved to [new state] in February of 1989. The husband hurt his back and could not help with the move and/or child care. Therefore, the patient was left to cope with a new living situation in a new city, care of a newborn infant, and her first experience in moving away from her family. The family reported that the patient made statements to the effect that she could do it all, and did not need to eat or sleep, and that she was a very strong person. Resultant to this situation, the patient began to distort and exaggerate her religious philosophies and books that she was reading, interpreting these as "special messages from God." The patient began to make statements that she had heard the voice of God and began exhibiting confused behaviors. She would stare at the sun, believing that she was getting certain communications from God.

She read a book about allergies, and based upon certain chapters of this book, she threw out all of the plastic in the home, including the baby's bassinet, cleaning supplies, and turned off the heat. Because the baby had no place of its own to sleep, the child then slept with the patient and her husband, significantly interrupting the patient's sleep pattern to the extent that she did not sleep for several days. Also, based upon her reading, she refused to eat or drink anything but spring water. She has lost 20 pounds in three weeks. The patient sang religious hymns repetitively and was found on a public street in her underwear, staring at the sun. At this time, three days prior to her admission, the husband returned to [home state] with the patient and his daughter in order to seek the support of the patient's parents and assistance in obtaining mental health services.

After going to the private hospital, Jenny was sent back to the state hospital for her "uncooperative attitude" regarding the administration of medications. These next excerpts are from the discharge summary from her second stay at the state hospital. It is during these 6 days that she went to court to try to avoid having to take antipsychotic medications.

Reason for Admission:

This 21 year old, white female was admitted on a Medical Certificate. She was transferred from [private hospital] because of her uncooperative behavior with the treatment. She was refusing to have any lab work done or comply with any medication. Before she was at [private hospital] she was at [state hospital]. Although she did go for a hearing and agreed to treatment, she did not cooperate when she went to [private hospital]. She has been for treatment. She has been having delusions.

Clinical Course:

The patient stayed on the Fourth Level until 4/18/89. She remained very uncooperative and guarded and paranoid. She was very much suspicious. She was very negative and was not responding to any questions. She was observed to be singing in the hallways and humming. She did not understand the need for treatment. She was approached for the physical examination and for the psychiatric evaluation almost every day. She did not cooperate very much except for the last few days. She was much more cooperative and did give some information. She provided that she had been acting very manic and hyperactive in the past. She agreed that she was doing some bizarre things. She has been scared and afraid and paranoid. Through the counseling she was willing to go to the private hospital and get treatment.

The next section is from the psychosocial history. The informants for this report are Jenny's parents. There is a great deal of overlap with the history reported at the time of first discharge. Some differences also provide additional information about her illness:

The patient is described as tending to be enthusiastic, generally does well at most things she attempts but tends to be "hard on herself if she finds herself falling short of her own expectations." She's considered to be very bright and creative, theatrically inclined and artistic. She enjoys being involved but tends to be very strong willed "not shy about expressing her opinions."

Although the family sees her emotional problems as starting on the day of daughter's delivery, the patient's obstetrician indicated that he thought he noticed manic symptoms approximately three weeks previously. [Note: He did not note these symptoms in her medical records, however.] The patient had planned on natural childbirth at [hospital name], in the birthing room, but at the time of the delivery became very angry when her doctor broke her waters and insisted on exercising certain hospital procedures which she objected to. She also was angry with her parents and husband for not backing her up, at the time of the birth there were five family members in the birthing room. The parents indicate that the patient was somewhat obsessed with having natural childbirth and that some of her expectations were unrealistic. The mother feels that she was not psychotic at the time of the birth, but did become so following her move to [another state]. The patient became even more inclined to believe what she read in various books, particularly being obsessed with a book on allergy, to the point she ran up considerable phone bills telling people to read the book then went on a three day fast, while nursing her baby. She started perceiving her husband as being evil and unclean because he works with computers and was not sympathetic to her expectations. It appears that her husband expressed some regrets at the idea of "never having a Big Mac or chocolate chip cookies again." She allegedly would not let her husband in the house on their anniversary because "God told me not to let you in." In several phone calls to her mother, she told her that "Satan is causing it."

ANALYSIS

The author of the psychosocial report apparently recognized that Jenny's illness had multiple causes. The report specifically mentions fatigue that was aggravated by and related to her mania, problems with social support brought on by her move to another state, and high expectations for herself as a wife and mother (wanting to be the best at everything). Further, the lack of sleep may have exacerbated any underlying condition caused by either a hormonal imbalance, history of allergies, or a combination of both (although this connection was never explored directly). Fasting may have resulted in a metabolic imbalance that, in combination with other factors, triggered the psychosis. The lack of social support in the new town also may have allowed her illness to progress as far as it did.

What is particularly interesting is the apparent lack of understanding about the role of Jenny's birth experience in her illness by both her family and the people treating her. They viewed her expectations as "unrealistic." According to Jenny, clinicians at the state hospital tended to focus on her birth experience, in some cases to the exclusion of all the other underlying factors. They focused on it while dismissing her feelings about it, as if naming her expectations as "unrealistic" would make her sense of disappointment and anger disappear. These issues and her perceptions of these events were important to her. Ironically, had her feelings been validated and had she been allowed to express them, her feelings of anger and disappointment could have dissipated. As it was, they continued to exert an influence. Jenny addressed her birth experience in a follow-up letter that she sent after reviewing a draft of the present volume's chapter on negative birth experiences. She also comments on how the trauma continued in the mental hospitals:

> It was so cool to read the Traumagenics Model, first in relation to my birth experience, and second, most importantly, to my hospitalization, which was 10x worse than my birth. "Powerlessness." (I was strapped to the four-point table for 2 ½ days!!) . . . I think you can tell that I experienced physical damage to a small degree, stigmatization somewhat, betrayal was the most intense of the four areas, and powerlessness definitely, although I *do* feel a great deal of satisfaction that I fought these ego-maniac doctors tooth and nail both during [my baby's] birth and again in refusing the drugs.
>
> I don't know that I'm in a position to critique the chapter, except on a personal basis as it related to me. All I can say is that it spoke to my soul and analytically broke down the areas of importance and organized them in such a way that as I read I found myself nodding in agreement and saying "Oh, *that* is what that emotion I experienced is called." It also totally added validity to my experience, which from most sides could be called the "ideal natural birth," but as you could hopefully pick up from my journal recording of the event, it did not go well from "my" perspective. And if my perspective doesn't count, whose does?
>
> Perception is everything! I strongly feel that because I was a probated patient to the mental hospital, my perceptions were significantly different from those of the other patients mostly because 90% of them signed themselves in. Where being locked up in a smoky, airless, pit of despair may have given some a sense of comfort and security (and some that I talked to expressed those exact sentiments), for me it was hell on earth.
>
> It was the same with [my baby's] birth. The high expectations for natural childbirth were always there, and I think that is why my Lamaze class was such a disappointment. And then when I read the Bradley materials three weeks before she was born and freaked out. My perceptions went from "I'll just roll with it and everything will work out" to "I'm going to have to fight to *make*

this happen the way I want." It wasn't the Bradley books that gave me my expectations. I think every woman expects and wants things to go smoothly. The materials simply empowered me to first decide what was important, second have the confidence to fight for it rather than passively agree, third know *how* to labor, and fourth just plain old go for it. I shudder to think how it would have been had I not got my hands on those books.

Being a Bradley teacher, I've heard doctors complain against natural childbirth saying that it builds unrealistic expectations and leads to PPD because their desires were not fulfilled. This ignorance-is-bliss mode is really scary. The fact that they used Scopolamine for so many years, a drug that helps people to forget, or at least blocks the conscious mind from remembering trauma (but it does not block pain), tells me it's not the women and their high expectations that are the problem. Knowledge is power and when we empower women to do what nature designed them to do, and then let them *do it*, what beauty and joy transpire! I love my doctor now, and he loves his Bradley couples because as he put it, "they are so prepared."

I know it would cramp many hospitals' style to just let a woman alone, with her husband to do her own thing. I don't *ever* see them doing that, but if they would, we really could have utopia with birth. I teach this analogy in my class. Comparing childbirth to swimming, the mother is the swimmer out there doing the work. The husband is the coach, encouraging. He's been with her all through the training, watching her nutrition, encouraging exercise, etc. . . . .And the doctor/hospital, they are the lifeguards watching, observing, staying back, but jumping in to save when deemed necessary. If hospitals could grasp this perspective we could really change things.

THE ROAD TO RECOVERY

Jenny's recovery from her postpartum illness was a lengthy process. At the time of this writing, almost 2 years had elapsed. After her first stay in the private mental hospital, she was transferred back to the state hospital for 6 days. During this time she went to court to avoid being forced to take antipsychotic medication. The account of her continuing recovery is taken from an interview conducted for this book:

During the 6 days back in the state mental hospital, I was literally a prisoner until I went to court. I had no friends, except for the other patients. Everyone was pressuring me. I called TV stations and reporters. One reporter was very supportive and wrote an article on postpartum depression. . . . While I was there, I was crazy. I'd sing patriotic songs and talk about my rights. During that time I was totally confused. I demanded a jury trial, which was my right. But they treated it like a joke. I wasn't a zombie. My sentence was 90 days, forced medications if necessary. When I heard that, my heart literally broke. I couldn't fight it anymore. Back at the hospital, my mom yelled at me for 3 hours. She said that I had to take the drugs and come home and take care of my baby. I finally couldn't fight anymore.

I went back to the private hospital and started on lithium and Stelazine. I started to self-destruct and overeat. They told me it would "fix" the chemical imbalance in my brain. I didn't know it [Stelazine] was a tranquilizer. When I started on the drugs, I was confused, couldn't finish a thought, tired (I slept 16-20 hours a day), and depressed. The drugs worked though. They stopped the mania and racing thoughts. I'm not against drugs, only the improper use of drugs. Once I complied, I could do what I wanted. I was totally cooperative and even warm to my doctor, doing everything he said.

After 2 weeks in the private hospital, she was released and stayed for 5 weeks at her parents' home. She then went home to her husband:

A big part of my recovery was going home to [new state] and facing my demons. I was worried about having no friends, about isolation. It was important to face what I was frightened of and being forced to be a mom again.

To help herself recover, she took her medications faithfully. She also began to put on weight and gained 50 pounds during that time. She started having severe PMS after coming home from the hospital. One psychiatrist told her she would be on lithium for the rest of her life. That news was devastating. She called Depression After Delivery (DAD) and got a referral for a new psychiatrist. She went on progesterone, which helped with her PMS, and stopped lithium, but she was still on Stelazine. She started on Prozac and got really depressed. She was hospitalized again and was suicidal. Another doctor took her off Stelazine, which helped, and doubled her dosage of Prozac.

She identified several activities as helping her recover. She started a support group for postpartum depression, was a DAD phone volunteer, and became a Bradley childbirth educator. "That was really important. Being around these happy couples who accepted me as a normal person." She had one 20-minute flashback about a year after her release from the hospital. "That was scary. I thought I had beaten it. I didn't go on lithium or back in the hospital. It helped not to emphasize it." A pivotal moment came when she read an article in *Newsweek* about Prozac. It was then that she decided to try to wean herself away from the medications:

> During that time, I was having highs and lows; really manic. I started looking for alternatives. During this time, I was obsessed with getting pregnant again to show I could do it right. I prayed. I discovered homeopathic, which cleanses the body. I discovered Chinese herbs. I feel this was from the Lord. Otherwise, I'd be on antidepressants again. It really helped. Going off of the drugs was like detox. I cried for a whole week. I think all the suppressed emotions of the last year came out.
>
> I went through all the stages of grief, especially grief itself. It was so healing to have this time. I gained an additional 50 pounds. I didn't understand. I couldn't figure out what was happening until I read a book on detox—this is part of it. I still had severe PMS. I became a hermit. I was still obsessed with becoming pregnant, and I was somewhat depressed. Spiritually, I was completely depressed—I didn't want to talk to God. But it was a healing time, a happy time. I started to feel again. I could sing, feel joy, enjoy [my baby], my husband.
>
> In January I began a weight loss program with Chinese herbs and lost 30 pounds. I've paid lots of attention to nutrition. I have a semi-vegetarian life-style. I eat organic foods and drink distilled water. I've had no drugs for over a year. I use homeopathics, do yoga, and exercise faithfully.

Jenny has identified six factors that helped her heal: (a) time to heal, (b) the support of her husband, (c) adequate nutrition (including fruits, vegetables, and dietary supplements), (d) grieving over her lost time with her daughter, (e) prayer of friends and family, and (f) having another baby (thus moving on with her life).

Overall, Jenny is philosophical about her experience and feels that good has come of it. She summarizes her feelings this way.

I don't regret that this happened. I don't feel bitter. I feel grateful to have had this experience. I didn't a year ago, but I do now. I feel empowered. Now I can empathize with other women, and I have placed myself in a key position to help other women. I don't know if I would have done this if I hadn't had this experience. I'd rather have had this experience than a normal easy birth. It uncluttered my life. It was the ultimate growth experience. I don't feel like I'm 23, I feel like I'm 50. I also feel that it was necessary. God allows things to happen to allow us to grow. Mental illness was not part of my plan, but it empowered me like nothing else could have to do what I needed to do.

NOTE

1. "Garments" are religious underclothing worn by Mormons.

SEVEN

Final Comments and Suggestions

Throughout this book we have offered suggestions about how you can help new mothers suffering from postpartum depression. In this chapter we make some final suggestions and offer an outline for prevention.

Be Open to a Variety of Possible Causes

As we have described in the last six chapters, the causes of postpartum illness are complex. Many women we have spoken with indicated that it was extremely frustrating when professionals made snap judgments about the causes of their depression without knowing the circumstances of their lives or really listening to them. Being told "Your expectations are too high" or "It's because you had a c-section" or some other pat answer can be extremely demoralizing if the women do not feel that the factor you mentioned is the cause of their distress. By listening carefully to what women say, you provide them with valuable support. Talking to women about a variety of possible causes lets them know that you are not approaching them with all the answers and that you see them as individuals. In addition, when women feel that you have really heard them, they are more likely to be open to your other suggestions.

Make Effective Use of Referrals

Your intervention with new mothers can encompass a wide variety of behaviors. In previous chapters we have described teaching specific behaviors to mothers or providing ongoing social support, which are two examples of active interventions. Your intervention may involve simply identifying the problem and making an appropriate referral. As we have indicated previously, making referrals to sources of help is an important service and may be the only one that you can realistically provide, given your length of contact with mothers and the constraints of your job.

When considering the types of referrals to make, it is best to offer a variety of treatment options, including support groups, psychiatrists, therapists, parent education groups, or simply places where women can go to meet other mothers. Some women find support groups to be very helpful, while others find them to be threatening or boring. Similarly, not every woman needs to be on antidepressants; they might benefit more from education, individual psychotherapy, or a combination of these. Contact mothers to whom you gave referrals to see whether a "good match" was made or whether she needs some other alternatives. Call Depression After Delivery (see the Appendix) or ask your colleagues for names of mental health professionals and support groups in your area that deal with postpartum illness. As a general rule we strongly recommend that you interview these people or assess groups yourself before you make referrals to them. After you have made a referral, we strongly encourage you to follow up with mothers to make sure they have made contact with your referral source. You might even consider making that initial contact yourself, especially if the mother appears too paralyzed by her depression to reach out for help.

When discussing referrals, the issue of cost often arises. As we indicated in Chapter 4, postpartum depression affects women of all socioeconomic levels, and low-income women are at even greater risk. Unfortunately, low-income women often lack access to adequate health care and are less likely to have as many treatment options as do middle-class women. A referral to a psychiatrist may not be realistic for a woman with no health insurance or whose insurance does not cover mental health services. It is for these women in particular that we make the following suggestions. Even as we make these suggestions, we realize that they fall far short of coordinated support efforts that women in many countries receive—and all women deserve. We also recognize that the suggestions may not be effective for women seriously affected by postpartum illness. Yet we have tried to provide suggestions that can be implemented within the limits of the present system.

In the Appendix are listed names of organizations that provide services for little or no cost. Many communities have local chapters of these organizations, where mothers can receive support and information. In addition, local chapters of these organizations often know of other sources of support within the community.

If you live in a community that lacks resources for new mothers, you might recommend several things. One short-term option is telephone support. Several organizations have toll-free numbers or telephone support people in various locations. This option is particularly helpful for crisis intervention but is not a long-term solution. Another option is a list of places where mothers can meet other mothers. Locate local parks, fast-food restaurants with play yards, neighborhood health clinics, or parks and recreation departments. Organizations such as the YMCA or the Salvation Army often have services for parents. Local churches may have play groups, respite day care, or discussion groups. Many of these services are not advertised but are known through word of mouth. The more of these types of volunteer programs you know about, the more options you will be able to offer.

Those suggestions are examples of what you can do for a mother right now. For a long-term solution to a lack of resources, you might consider starting a support program or parent-mentoring program yourself. Local charitable or fraternal organizations or hospitals might be willing to sponsor such an effort by providing small grants, administrative support, or a location for meetings. In addition, the National Resource Center for Family Support Programs can provide information and training for professionals who wish to start a family support program. Further, the National Resource Center on Family Based Services also offers information on program development, training, and program evaluation for family support programs (see the Appendix). Both of these organizations can help you improve the level of support for new mothers in your community.

The Road to Recovery Can Be Long

As Jenny indicated in the previous chapter, recovery from postpartum illness can take months or even years. The prognosis for recovery is good but never instant—even with medications. Without discouraging women, you may want to prepare them for the fact that recovery is a process. As such, it can take a long time. Joanne and Karen both describe how their depressions changed their lives:

There were lots of positive things [about my depression]. I was forced to evaluate how I live life. . . . Everything fit in my world prior to that. When the depression hit, every strategy I had for living life fell apart. Everything turned upside down. My capacity to enjoy life is much better now. Trusting the Lord, what it means to love others and be compassionate. When I can't fix myself and the world, I have to rethink what is important and what is my value based on. I had to evaluate my past. There were some painful things there that I had to work on, that I had swept under the carpet. I've turned out to be very grateful. The Lord used this to rattle my cage. At the time, I thought it would be better to have cancer. At least that's something tangible. I must admit that although there are many wonderful changes in my life because of experiencing depression, I would never want to go through it again. My postpartum experiences are less than desirable. I find I still feel somewhat disappointed at the limited resources available to women from the medical profession. I occasionally tend to feel less womanly for not having a wonderful experience with my babies. And I feel handicapped that having another baby would take so much strength and courage, with so little support available [Joanne].

Once you are past a certain amount of months postpartum, people don't want to talk about it anymore. It's like you have an ego problem or something. But I need to talk about it. It's been too important of an experience for me not to talk about it. It's changed my life. . . . In some ways, it was a good experience to have. It's totally changed my outlook, the way I look at other women [Karen].

The stories of these two women demonstrate the amount of upheaval that postpartum depression can create in a woman's life. Even though their experiences differ, both have become actively involved in helping other women recover from postpartum illness. Their stories give a more realistic perspective on recovery.

Involve Women in Their Own Prevention Efforts

As we have described previously, mothers in western cultures receive little or no preparation for the postpartum period, as all attention is focused on preparing them for labor and delivery. To a certain extent, the focus on labor and delivery is needed because women may not be psychologically prepared for the reality of birth. Some anticipatory guidance is necessary. It is just as important to prepare women for the emotional and physiological changes they might experience during the puerperium.

In many circles people dread informing pregnant women about the possibility of postpartum depression for fear of "worrying" them. Although it is important for women to have information about postpartum depression, they are frequently not given enough to be of use. For example, women are generally not given any information about what they can do about postpartum depression (other than a vague "Come see us if you experience these symptoms") or what they can do to prevent it.

In an ideal world women would receive adequate support throughout the postpartum period and beyond. Panuthos and Romeo (1984) indicated that 250 countries throughout the world do a more effective job of providing postpartum support than that provided for new mothers in the United States. Mothers in other countries are provided with practical assistance and support while they recover from birth and learn how to be mothers. In contrast, many American mothers have no such apprentice period and must fully function as mothers by the time they leave the hospital. Although some individual hospitals and communities have attempted to alleviate this problem, it may be many years before these types of services are available to all mothers.

Until all mothers receive support services, we encourage you to involve women in their own prevention efforts. The childbirth education class may be the most effective vehicle for prevention efforts. If you are a childbirth educator, consider dedicating at least a few hours of your childbirth education class to the postpartum period, during which time you can review with mothers and fathers some of the physiological and emotional changes that they are likely to experience. Provide information on what they can do to survive the postpartum period, and consider including information on diet, exercise, parenting, child care information, and social support.

Labor and delivery are physical events that can physically deplete women and make them more vulnerable to depression. A nutritious diet is essential to recovery from childbirth (Panuthos & Romeo, 1984). A diet high in carbohydrates will boost energy and increase levels of serotonin in the brain, both of which may decrease the likelihood of depression (Wurtman & Wurtman, 1989). It is easy to ignore proper nutrition once the baby is born, and yet adequate nutritional intake can make a difference in the mother's postpartum adjustment. Providing women and their partners with basic nutritional information, including guidelines on the amounts of food they should eat, may make them more likely to eat a well-balanced diet. A simple food diary or checklist also might help women monitor their daily intake.

Your preparation training also should include a component that helps mothers feel more competent as parents. Classes for mothers in the hospital are a helpful beginning, but postpartum education is important too. You can provide mothers with a list of classes, groups, or visiting nurses that provide child care information in the event they need further information after leaving the hospital.

Breast-feeding difficulties can be a source of distress for many new mothers. Prenatal information on breast-feeding is helpful, but perhaps more important is information on sources of postnatal support. Women who encounter difficulties and who have no support are more likely to discontinue breast-feeding. This could add to their feelings that they are less than adequate as mothers.

A final component involves women's sources of social support. Many of the mothers we spoke with indicated that they were truly surprised by how isolated and abandoned they felt once they had their babies. One somewhat touchy issue that you might address is the potential role of the woman's own mother. Many women automatically assume that they will have their mother (or other female relative) stay with them after the baby is born. Although a woman's mother can be a source of tremendous help, she can also be a problem, especially if she is critical or attempts to take over in baby care (thus undermining the woman's confidence). Women should assess realistically whether their mothers or other family members will be helpful or detrimental in those first postpartum days. Women who decide that they do not want their relatives to be there initially can suggest a visit a few weeks later, once they feel more confident with their babies.

It is also generally helpful for women to have friends with babies or small children. If a mother does not know many other people with small children, you may need to brainstorm with her about where she could meet other mothers with whom she might have something in common and who will be supportive of her.

If you have an opportunity to speak with the father of the baby, remember that he can be a very important source of support. Encourage him to pay extra attention to his partner *after* the baby is born because everyone else's attention will be focused on the baby. Suggest that he do anything he can to make her feel special and important. And, if at all possible, strongly encourage him to take some time off of work. Many men do just the opposite after a baby is born and *increase* the amount of hours they work, because they feel pressure to be "super-providers." They may not realize how important their emotional support will be to their partners until you tell them. Realize too that the fathers need support. In your preparation of mothers do not forget the fathers. They also will experience many emotional changes and should also be encouraged to seek support.

Conclusion

We hope the information presented in this book is of use to you. We strongly encourage you to get involved in the lives of new mothers. You are in a position to make an important contribution to the well-being of mothers, their babies, and the rest of their families. We wish you success in this important work.

Locating Resources Within Your Community

Much of your work in intervening in cases of postpartum depression will involve making appropriate referrals to services and resources within your community. The purpose of this section is to help you prepare a list of such services.

The first place to start is with local hospitals. Find out what services they have for new mothers, including classes, mental health services, support groups, services for parents of sick or premature infants, postpartum care, and postpartum exercise. Also look in your local yellow pages under "Social Services," "Women's Health," "Family Planning," or similar categories to find other services. Agencies such as the YWCA/YMCA, Salvation Army, Family Service Association, Department of Social Services, the local children's hospital, or Jewish Family and Children's Services often have a wealth of services and referral sources (many of these are free or low cost). Other resources that you should try to locate are mental health services for women suffering from postpartum depression (Depression After Delivery can help you find these) and 24-hour hot lines that women can call for support, information, assistance with their babies, and in general. It may take some investigative work on your part to locate this information, because centralized referral sources are rare. Further, we suggest that you call all the places that might have services and screen the agency personnel you speak with. List only services that are courteous on the telephone, are prompt at returning calls, and seem to offer services that you feel would be helpful to mothers. Women suffering from postpartum depression do not need or deserve the added stress of dealing with a rude agency or one that does not do what it says it will do.

Once you have located this information, consider printing up booklets to give to mothers. If you cannot do that, develop a list for your own use so that you can make referrals when the need arises. You may want to organize the information under the following categories (modifying them to fit the resources available in your community) and repeat entries if they fall under more than one category:

Breast-feeding
   Education
   Support
Cesarean sections
   c-section support
   Prepared cesarean classes
   VBAC classes
Child care referrals
Depression
Education
   Child care preparation/parenting
   Infant safety
   Prenatal
   Prepared childbirth
Exercise
   Prenatal
   Postpartum
Maternity and children's clothing (including consignment shops)
Medical referrals
New-mother support (including support groups and household assistance)
Nutrition (including WIC and agencies that provide nutrition education)
Postpartum care
Special needs' babies
   Handicapped
   Premature

Twins

Stress (including numbers for hot lines)

Teen mothers (list services especially designed for teen mothers)

To aid your process of discovering local resources, the following list of national organizations can provide information and referrals to services within your community.

ARCH: The National Resource Center for Crisis Nurseries and Respite Care Services

The mission of this organization is to provide support to service providers through training, technical assistance, evaluation and research. It also has an information center that provides access to local, state, and national resources.

Chapel Hill Training-Outreach Project
800 Eastowne Drive, Suite 105
Chapel Hill, NC 27514
(800) 473-1727

ChildHelp USA

24-hour hotline for victims of abuse, abusers, or those wishing to report abuse. Also offers referrals to local resources, literature, and crisis counseling.

6463 Independence Avenue
Woodland Hills, CA 91367
(800) 4-A-CHILD

C/SEC (Cesarean/Support, Education, Concern)

Provides information and support for those who have had cesarean sections, and referrals to local support groups. It also has information on c-section recovery, cesarean prevention, and VBAC.

22 Forest Road
Framingham, MA 01701
(508) 877-8266

Depression After Delivery, National

DAD has information on postpartum depression and psychosis, and referrals to local support groups, psychiatrists, and phone volunteers.

P.O. Box 1282
Morrisville, PA 19067
(215) 295-3994

Federation for Children With Special Needs

This national help organization offers networking and training for parents caring for children with special needs.

95 Berkeley Street, Suite 104
Boston, MA 02116
(617) 482-2915

International Cesarean Awareness Network (I CAN)

A nationwide, volunteer-run, peer support organization. I CAN's priority is woman-to-woman support, particularly around the emotional issues associated with cesarean birth. It also provides information.

P.O. Box 152
Syracuse, NY 13210
(315) 424-1942

La Leche League International

A well-known organization for support and information for breast-feeding mothers. Provides lactation consultation via telephone (9 a.m.-3 p.m. CST), breast-feeding information, and referrals to local chapters.

9616 Minneapolis Avenue
Franklin Park, IL 60131
(708) 455-7730
(800) LaLeche

National Down Syndrome Congress

Support and information for parents of children with Down syndrome.

1800 Dempster Street
Park Ridge, IL 60068
(708) 823-7550
(800) 232-6372

National Foundation—March of Dimes Birth Defects Foundation

Information and referral source.

1275 Mamaroneck Avenue
White Plains, NY 10605
(914) 428-7100

National Information Center for Children and Youth With Handicaps

This organization provides information regarding handicaps for children up to age 21. It also has a national toll-free number and individuals in each state who can help locate assistance in your local area.

P.O. Box 1492
Washington, DC 20013
(800) 999-5599

National Organization of Mothers of Twins Clubs, Inc.

An organization with many local chapters aimed at helping and supporting parents of twins (and other multiple births).

P.O. Box 23188
Albuquerque, NM 87192-1188
(505) 275-0955

National Resource Center on Family Based Services

An organization that provides training and program evaluation for family support programs.

University of Iowa School of Social Work
112 North Hall
Iowa City, IA 52242
(319) 335-2200

National Resource Center for Family Support Programs

A membership organization that can refer parents to local support groups and can provide training for professionals who wish to start their own family support program.

200 South Michigan Avenue, Suite 1520
Chicago, IL 60604
(312) 341-0900

National Women's Health Network

A national information clearinghouse and lobbying group on issues related to women's health. It has information on cesarean birth, postpartum depression, depression in general, and antidepressant medications.

1325 G Street NW
Washington, DC 20005
(202) 347-1140

Parents Anonymous, National

Help for parents who have abused their children or who are afraid that they might do so. Call the main office for information on local chapters and crisis lines.

520 South Lafayette Park Place, Suite 316
Los Angeles, CA 90057
(213) 388-6685
(800) 421-0353

Postpartum Support International

An umbrella organization for other groups specializing in postpartum depression. It is a referral network and can offer referrals worldwide. It also offers training for professionals and information.

927 North Kellogg Avenue
Santa Barbara, CA 93111
(805) 967-7636

Santa Barbara Birth Resource Center

Referrals to organizations throughout the United States. Send a self-addressed stamped envelope for a brochure listing their publications, including low-cost pamphlets on postpartum depression written in both English and Spanish.

1525 Santa Barbara Street
Santa Barbara, CA 93101
(805) 966-4545

References

Abramson, L. Y., Seligman, M. E. P., & Teasdale, J. D. (1978). Learned helplessness in humans: Critique and reformulation. *Journal of Abnormal Psychology, 87*, 49-74.

Adler, T. (1991a). Therapy may best treat panic disorder. *APA Monitor, 22*, 10.

Adler, T. (1991b). Depression, surroundings linked. *APA Monitor, 22*, 16-17.

Affleck, G., Tennen, H., Rowe, J., Roscher, B., & Walker, L. (1989). Effects of formal support on mothers' adaptation to the hospital-to-home transition of high-risk infants: The benefits and costs of helping. *Child Development, 60*, 488-501.

Affonso, D. D. (1977). "Missing pieces"—A study of postpartum feelings. *Birth and the Family Journal, 4*, 159-164.

Affonso, D. D. (1979). Risks in puerperal adaptation. In A. L. Clark, D. D. Affonso, with T. R. Harris (Eds.), *Childbearing: A nursing perspective* (2nd ed., pp. 729-744). Philadelphia: F. A. Davis.

Affonso, D. D., & Arizmendi, T. G. (1986). Disturbances in post-partum adaptation and depressive symptomatology. *Journal of Psychosomatic Obstetrics and Gynaecology, 5*, 15-32.

Affonso, D. D., & Stichler, J. F. (1978). Exploratory study of women's reactions to having a cesarean birth. *Birth and the Family Journal, 5*, 88-94.

Affonso, D. D., & Walpole, J. (1979). Management of pain associated with labor and birth. In A. L. Clark, D. D. Affonso, with T. R. Harris (Eds.), *Childbearing: A nursing perspective* (2nd ed., pp. 417-450). Philadelphia: F. A. Davis.

Ainsworth, M. D. S. (1979). Infant-mother attachment. *American Psychologist, 34*, 932-937.

American Psychiatric Association. (1980). *Diagnostic and Statistical Manual, III.* Washington, DC: Author.

Atkinson, H. (1985). *Women and fatigue.* New York: Pocket.

Atkinson, J. H., Ingram, R. E., Kremer, E. F., & Saccuzzo, D. P. (1986). MMPI subgroups and affective disorder in chronic pain patients. *Journal of Nervous and Mental Disease, 174*, 408-413.

Balchin, P. (1975). The midwife and puerperal psychosis. *Midwife, Health Visitor, and Community Nurse, 11*, 41-43.

Barnett, B., & Parker, G. (1985). Professional and non-professional intervention for highly anxious primiparous mothers. *British Journal of Psychiatry, 146*, 287-293.

Bendersky, M., & Lewis, M. (1986). The impact of birth order on mother-infant interactions in preterm and sick infants. *Journal of Developmental and Behavioral Pediatrics, 7*, 242-246.

Bennett, H. (1990, Fall). Support for new mothers. *Health Notes*, p. 6.

Blumberg, N. L. (1980). Effects of neonatal risk, maternal attitude, and cognitive style on early postpartum adjustment. *Journal of Abnormal Psychology, 89*, 139-150.

Boukydis, C. F. Z., Lester, B. M., & Hoffman, J. (1987). Parenting and social support networks for parents of preterm and fullterm infants. In C.F.Z. Boukydis (Ed.), *Research on support for parents and infants in the postnatal period* (pp. 61-83). Norwood, NJ: Ablex.

Bradley, C. F., Ross, S. E., & Warnyca, J. (1983). A prospective study of mothers' attitudes and feelings following cesarean and vaginal births. *Birth, 10*, 79-83.

Brazelton, T. B., Tronick, E., Adamson, L., Als, H., & Wise, S. (1975). Early mother-infant reciprocity. In M. Hofer (Ed.), *Parent-infant interaction* (pp. 137-145). Amsterdam: Elsevier.

Bridge, L. R., Little, B. C., Hayworth, J., Dewhurst, J., & Priest, R. G. (1985). Psychometric ante-natal predictors of post-natal depressed mood. *Journal of Psychosomatic Research, 29*, 325-331.

Buss, A. H., & Plomin, R. (1975). *A temperament theory of personality development*. New York: John Wiley.

Butler, J., & Leonard, B. E. (1986). Post-partum depression and the effect of nomifensine treatment. *International Clinical Psychopharmacology, 1*, 244-252.

Campbell, S. B., Cohn, J. F., Flanagan, C., Popper, S., & Meyers, T. (1992). Course and correlates of postpartum depression during the transition to parenthood. *Development and Psychopathology, 4*, 29-47.

Campos, J., Bartlett, K. C., Lamb, M. E., Goldsmith, H. H., & Stenberg, C. (1983). Socioemotional development. In P. Mussen (Ed.), *Handbook of child psychology* (Vol. II, 4th ed., pp. 784-915). New York: John Wiley.

Capuzzi, C. (1989). Maternal attachment to handicapped infants and the relationship to social support. *Research in Nursing and Health, 12*, 161-167.

Chalmers, B. E., & Chalmers, B. M. (1986). Post-partum depression: A revised perspective. *Journal of Psychosomatic Obstetrics and Gynaecology, 5*, 93-105.

Chess, S., & Thomas, A. (1977). Temperamental individuality from childhood to adolescence. *Journal of Child Psychiatry, 16*, 218-226.

Clark, A. L. (1979a). Prematurity. In A. L. Clark, D. D. Affonso, with T. R. Harris (Eds.), *Childbearing: A nursing perspective* (2nd ed., pp. 939-948). Philadelphia: F. A. Davis.

Clark, A. L. (1979b). Abnormality. In A. L. Clark, D. D. Affonso, with T. R. Harris (Eds.), *Childbearing: A nursing perspective* (2nd ed., pp. 961-970). Philadelphia: F. A. Davis.

Cogill, S. R., Caplan, H. L., Alexandra, H., Robson, K. M., & Kumar, R. (1986). Impact of maternal postnatal depression on cognitive development of young children. *British Medical Journal, 292*, 1165-1167.

Cowan, C. P., & Cowan, P. A. (1987). A preventive intervention for couples becoming parents. In C. F. Z. Boukydis (Ed.), *Research on support for parents and infants in the postnatal period* (pp. 225-252). Norwood, NJ: Ablex.

Cox, J. L. (1988). Childbirth as a life event: Sociocultural aspects of postnatal depression. *Acta Psychiatrica Scandanavica Supplement, 344,* 75-83.

Cox, J. L., Connor, Y., & Kendell, R. E. (1982). Prospective study of the psychiatric disorders of childbirth. *British Journal of Psychiatry, 140,* 111-117.

Cox, J. L., Holden, J. M., & Sagovsky, R. (1987). Detection of postnatal depression: Development of the 10-item Edinburgh Postnatal Depression Scale. *British Journal of Psychiatry, 150,* 782-786.

Cranley, M. S., Hedahl, K. J., & Pegg, S. H. (1983). Women's perceptions of vaginal and cesarean deliveries. *Nursing Research, 32,* 10-15.

Crnic, K., & Greenberg, M. (1987). Maternal stress, social support, and coping: Influences on the early mother-infant relationship. In C. F. Z. Boukydis (Ed.), *Research on support for parents and infants in the postnatal period* (pp. 25-41). Norwood, NJ: Ablex.

Crnic, K. A., Greenberg, M. T., & Slough, N. M. (1986). Early stress and social support influences on mothers' and high-risk infants' functioning in late infancy. *Infant Mental Health Journal, 7,* 19-33.

Crockenberg, S. (1981). Infant irritability, mother responsiveness, and social support influences on the security of infant attachment. *Child Development, 52,* 857-865.

Crockenberg, S. B. (1987). Support for adolescent mothers during the postnatal period: Theory and practice. In C. F. Z. Boukydis (Ed.), *Research on support for parents and infants in the postnatal period* (pp. 3-24). Norwood, NJ: Ablex.

Crockenberg, S., & McCluskey, K. (1986). Change in maternal behavior during the baby's first year of life. *Child Development, 57,* 746-753.

Culp, R. E., & Osofsky, H. J. (1989). Effects of cesarean delivery on parental depression, marital adjustment, and mother-infant interaction. *Birth, 16,* 53-57.

Cutrona, C. E. (1983). Causal attributions and perinatal depression. *Journal of Abnormal Psychology, 92,* 161-172.

Cutrona, C. E. (1984). Social support and stress in the transition to parenthood. *Journal of Abnormal Psychology, 93,* 378-390.

Cutrona, C. E., & Troutman, B. R. (1986). Social support, infant temperament, and parenting self-efficacy: A mediational model of postpartum depression. *Child Development, 57,* 1507-1518.

Dalton, K. (1971). Prospective study into puerperal depression. *British Journal of Psychiatry, 118,* 689-692.

Dalton, K. (1985). Progesterone prophylaxis used successfully in postnatal depression. *The Practitioner, 229,* 507-508.

Davidson, J. R. T. (1972). Postpartum mood change in Jamaican women: A description and discussion on its significance. *British Journal of Psychiatry, 121,* 659-663.

Davidson, J., & Robertson, E. (1985). A follow-up study of post-partum illness, 1946-1978. *Acta Psychiatrica Scandanavica, 71,* 451-457.

Dix, C. (1985). *The new mother syndrome.* New York: Pocket.

Donovan, W. L., & Leavitt, L. A. (1989). Maternal self-efficacy and infant attachment: Integrating physiology, perceptions, and behavior. *Child Development, 60,* 460-472.

Donovan, W. L., Leavitt, L. A., & Walsh, R. O. (1990). Maternal self-efficacy: Illusory control and its effect on susceptibility to learned helplessness. *Child Development, 61*, 1638-1647.

Durrett, M. E., Otaki, M., & Richards, P. (1984). Attachment and the mother's perception of support from the father. *International Journal of Behavioral Development, 7*, 167-176.

Eisenberg, A., Murkoff, H. E., & Hathaway, S. E. (1989). *What to expect the first year.* New York: Workman.

Erb, L., Hill, G., & Houston, D. (1983). A survey of parents' attitudes toward their cesarean births in Manitoba hospitals. *Birth, 10*, 85-92.

Feksi, A., Harris, B., Walker, R. F., Riad-Fahmy, D., & Newcomb, R. G. (1984). "Maternity blues" and hormone levels in saliva. *Journal of Affective Disorders, 6*, 351-355.

Field, T. (1992). Infants of depressed mothers. *Development and Psychopathology, 4*, 49-66.

Figley, C. R. (1986). Traumatic stress: The role of the family and social support system. In C. R. Figley (Ed.), *Trauma and its wake: Vol. II. Traumatic stress theory, research, and intervention* (pp. 39-54). New York: Bruner/Mazel.

Finkelhor, D. (1987). The trauma of child sexual abuse: Two models. *Journal of Interpersonal Violence, 2*, 348-366.

Fischer-Fay, F. A., Goldberg, S., Simmons, R., & Levison, H. (1988). Chronic illness and infant-mother attachment: Cystic fibrosis. *Journal of Developmental and Behavioral Pediatrics, 9*, 266-270.

Frodi, A., Bridges, L., & Shonk, S. (1989). Maternal correlates of infant temperament ratings and of infant-mother attachment: A longitudinal study. *Infant Mental Health Journal, 10*, 273-289.

Frommer, E. A., & O'Shea, G. (1973). Antenatal identification of women liable to have problems in managing their infants. *British Journal of Psychiatry, 123*, 149-156.

Gardner, D. L. (1991). Fatigue in postpartum women. *Applied Nursing Research, 4*, 57-62.

Gardner, D. L., & Campbell, B. (1991). Assessing postpartum fatigue. *MCN, 14*, 264-266.

Garel, M., Lelong, N., & Kaminski, M. (1987). Psychological consequences of caesarean childbirth in primiparas. *Journal of Psychosomatic Obstetrics and Gynecology, 6*, 197-209.

Gildenberg, P. L. (1984). Management of chronic pain. *Applied Neurophysiology, 47*, 157-170.

Goer, H. (1991, November). Not "just" another way to have a baby. *Baby Talk*, pp. 34-35.

Goldsmith, H. H., Bradshaw, D. L., & Rieser-Danner, L. A. (1986). Temperament as a potential developmental influence on attachment. In J. V. Lerner & R. M. Lerner (Eds.), *Temperament and social interaction during infancy and childhood: New directions for child development* (No. 3, pp. 5-34). San Francisco: Jossey-Bass.

Gotlib, I. H., Whiffen, V. E., Wallace, P. M., & Mount, J. H. (1991). Prospective investigation of postpartum depression: Factors involved in onset and recovery. *Journal of Abnormal Psychology, 100*, 122-132.

Hapgood, C. C., Elkind, G. S., & Wright, J. J. (1988). Maternity blues: Phenomena and relationship to later postpartum depression. *Australian and New Zealand Journal of Psychiatry, 22*, 299-306.

Harris, B., Fung, H., Johns, S., Kologlu, M., Bhatti, R., McGregor, A. M., Richards, C. J., & Hall, R. (1989). Transient postpartum thyroid dysfunction and postnatal depression. *Journal of Affective Disorders, 17,* 243-249.

Hayslip, C. C., Fein, H. G., O'Donnell, V. M., Friedman, D. S., Klein, T. A., & Smallridge, R. C. (1988). The value of serum antimicrosomal antibody testing in screening for symptomatic postpartum thyroid dysfunction. *American Journal of Obstetrics and Gynecology, 159,* 203-209.

Hoffman, Y., & Drotar, D. (1991). The impact of postpartum depressed mood on mother-infant interaction: Like mother like baby? *Infant Mental Health Journal, 12,* 65-80.

Holden, J. M., Sagovsky, R., & Cox, J. L. (1989). Counselling in a general practice setting: Controlled study of health visitor intervention in treatment of postnatal depression. *British Medical Journal, 298,* 223-226.

Hopkins, J., Marcus, M., & Campbell, S. B. (1984). Postpartum depression: A critical review. *Psychological Bulletin, 95,* 498-515.

Horowitz, M. J., & Kaltreider, N. B. (1979). Brief therapy of the stress response syndrome. *Psychiatric Clinics of North America, 2,* 365-377.

Hotchner, T. (1988). *Childbirth and marriage.* New York: Avon.

Howze, D. C., & Kotch, J. B. (1984). Disentangling life events, stress and social support: Implications for the primary prevention of child abuse and neglect. *Child Abuse and Neglect, 8,* 401-409.

Ifabumuyi, O. I., & Akindele, M. O. (1985). Post-partum mental illness in northern Nigeria. *Acta Psychiatrica Scandinavica, 72,* 63-68.

Janoff-Bulman, R. (1985). The aftermath of victimization: Rebuilding shattered assumptions. In C. R. Figley (Ed.), *Trauma and its wake: The study and treatment of post-traumatic stress disorder* (pp. 15-35). New York: Bruner/Mazel.

Jarvis, P. A., Myers, B. J., & Creasey, G. L. (1989). The effects of infants' illness on mothers' interactions with prematures at 4 and 8 months. *Infant Behavior and Development, 12,* 25-35.

Kalfus, M., & Shaffer, G. (1990, September 22). Newport woman jumps to her death at hotel. *Orange County Register,* p. B1.

Kantor, G. K. (1978). Addicted mother, addicted baby—A challenge to health care providers. *Maternal Child Nursing, 3,* 281-289.

Kellner, R., Buckman, M. T., Fava, M., Fava, G. A., & Mastrogiacomo, I. (1984). Prolactin, aggression and hostility: A discussion of recent studies. *Psychiatric Developments, 2,* 131-138.

Kendell, R. E., Mackenzie, W. E., West, C., McGuire, R. J., & Cox, J. L. (1984). Day-to-day mood changes after childbirth: Further data. *British Journal of Psychiatry, 145,* 620-625.

Kendell, R. E., McGuire, R. J., Connor, J., & Cox, J. L. (1981). Mood changes in the first three weeks after childbirth. *Journal of Affective Disorders, 3,* 317-326.

Kennerley, H., & Gath, D. (1986). Maternity blues reassessed. *Psychiatric Developments, 1,* 1-17.

Kinard, E. M. (1990, October). *Depression and social support in mothers of abused children.* Paper presented at the annual meetings of the American Public Health Association, New York.

Kitzinger, S. (1975). The fourth trimester? *Midwife, Health Visitor, and Community Nurse, 11,* 118-121.

Kitzinger, S. (1987). *Your baby, your way: Making pregnancy decisions and birth plans.* New York: Pantheon.

Klein, M. J. A. (1990). The home health nurse clinician's role in prevention of nonorganic failure to thrive. *Journal of Pediatric Nursing, 5,* 129-135.

Knight, R. G., & Thirkettle, J. A. (1987). The relationship between expectations of pregnancy and birth, and transient depression in the immediate postpartum period. *Journal of Psychosomatic Research, 31,* 351-357.

Kroetsch, P., & Shamoian, C. A. (1983). Pain and depression. *Journal of Psychiatric Treatment and Evaluation, 5,* 417-420.

Lachnit, C. (1990, May 24). Appeals court won't order retrial in postpartum psychosis killing. *Orange County Register,* p. B1.

Lahey, B. B. (1992). *Psychology* (4th ed.). Dubuque, IA: William C. Brown.

Leathe, M. (1987, Fall). Postpartum depression. *Mothering,* pp. 72-77.

Levitt, M. J., Weber, R. A., & Clark, M. C. (1986). Social network relationships as sources of maternal support and well-being. *Developmental Psychology, 22,* 310-316.

Levy, V. (1987). The maternity blues in postpartum and post-operative women. *British Journal of Psychiatry, 151,* 368-372.

Lewis, M., & Lee-Painter, S. (1974). An interactional approach to the mother-infant dyad. In M. Lewis & L. A. Rosenblum (Eds.), *The effect of the infant on its caregiver* (pp. 21-47). New York: John Wiley.

Liebman, B. (1990). PMS: Proof or promises? *Nutrition Action Health Letter, 17,* 5-7.

Lindy, J. D. (1986). An outline for the psychoanalytic psychotherapy of post-traumatic stress disorder. In C. R. Figley (Ed.), *Trauma and its wake: Vol. II. Traumatic stress theory, research, and intervention* (pp. 195-212). New York: Bruner/Mazel.

Luce, G. G. (1966). *Current research on sleep and dreams* (Public Health Service Publication No. 1389). Washington, DC: Public Health Service.

Lyons-Ruth, K., Connell, D. B., Grunebaum, H. U., & Botein, S. (1990). Infants at social risk: Maternal depression and family support services as mediators of infant development and security of attachment. *Child Development, 61,* 85-98.

Macey, T. J., Harmon, R. J., & Easterbrooks, M. A. (1987). Impact of premature birth on the development of the infant in the family. *Journal of Consulting and Clinical Psychology, 55,* 846-852.

Mandell, M., & Scanlon, L. W. (1979). *Dr. Mandell's 5-day allergy relief system.* New York: Pocket.

Manly, P. C., McMahon, R. J., Bradley, C. F., & Davidson, P. O. (1982). Depressive attributional style and depression following childbirth. *Journal of Abnormal Psychology, 91,* 245-254.

Marut, J. S., & Mercer, R. T. (1979). Comparison of primiparas' perceptions of vaginal and cesarean births. *Nursing Research, 28,* 260-266.

McCormack, P. (1991, July). Here's papa. *Parenting,* pp. 64-67.

McGrath, E., Keita, G. P., Strickland, B. R., & Russo, N. F. (1990). *Women and depression: Risk factors and treatment issues.* Washington, DC: American Psychological Association.

Moore, D. J. (1990, April). Why so blue? *Baby Talk,* pp. 34-35.

Mueller, C. (1985). On the nosology of postpartum psychoses. *Psychopathology, 18,* 181-184.

Naylor, A. (1982). Premature mourning and failure to mourn: Their relationship to conflict between mothers and intellectually normal children. *American Journal of Orthopsychiatry, 52*, 679-687.

Oakley, A. (1980). *Women confined.* Oxford: Martin Robertson.

Oakley, A. (1983). Social consequences of obstetric technology: The importance of measuring "soft" outcomes. *Birth, 10*, 99-108.

Ogier, J. (1982, April/May). Rebirthing of a natural act. *Whole Life Times,* pp. 25-27.

O'Hara, M. W. (1986). Social support, life events, and depression during pregnancy and the puerperium. *Archives of General Psychiatry, 43*, 569-573.

O'Hara, M. W. (1987). Post-partum "blues," depression, and psychosis: A review. Special issue: Maternal development during reproduction. *Journal of Psychosomatic Obstetrics and Gynaecology, 7*, 205-227.

O'Hara, M. W., Neunaber, D. J., & Zekoski, M. (1984). A prospective study of postpartum depression: Prevalence, course and predictive factors. *Journal of Abnormal Psychology, 93*, 158-171.

O'Hara, M. W., Rehm, L. P., & Campbell, S. B. (1982). Predicting depressive symptomatology: Cognitive-behavioral models of postpartum depression. *Journal of Abnormal Psychology, 91*, 457-461.

O'Hara, M. W., Rehm, L. P., & Campbell, S. B. (1983). Postpartum depression: A role for social network and life stress variables. *Journal of Nervous Disorders, 171*, 336-341.

O'Hara, M. W., Schlechte, J. A., Lewis, D. A., & Varner, M. W. (1991). Controlled prospective study of postpartum mood disorders: Psychological, environmental, and hormonal variables. *Journal of Abnormal Psychology, 100*, 63-73.

Padawer, J. A., Fagan, C., Janoff-Bulman, R., Strickland, B. R., & Chorowski, M. (1988). Women's psychological adjustment following emergency cesarean versus vaginal delivery. *Psychology of Women's Quarterly, 12*, 25-34.

Panuthos, C., & Romeo, C. (1984). *Ended beginnings: Healing childbearing losses.* New York: Bergin & Garvey.

Parke, R., & Tinsley, B. J. (1987). Fathers as agents and recipients of support in the postnatal period. In C. F. Z. Boukydis (Ed.), *Research on support for parents and infants in the postnatal period* (pp. 84-113). Norwood, NJ: Ablex.

Paykel, E. S., Emms, E. M., Fletcher, J., & Rassaby, E. S. (1980). Life events and social support in puerperal depression. *British Journal of Psychiatry, 136*, 339-346.

Pitt, B. (1968). Atypical depression following childbirth. *British Journal of Psychiatry, 114*, 1325-1335.

Pitt, B. (1973). Maternity blues. *British Journal of Psychiatry, 122*, 431-433.

Polansky, N. A., Gaudin, J. M., Ammons, P. W., & Davis, K. B. (1985). The psychological ecology of the neglectful mother. *Child Abuse and Neglect, 9*, 265-275.

Rathus, S. A. (1991). *Essentials of psychology* (3rd ed.). Fort Worth, TX: Holt, Rinehart and Winston.

Rieser-Danner, L. A., Roggman, L., & Langlois, J. H. (1987). Infant attractiveness and perceived temperament in the prediction of attachment classification. *Infant Mental Health Journal, 8*, 144-155.

Roediger, H. L., Rushton, J. P., Capaldi, E. D., & Paris, S. G. (1986). *Psychology* (2nd ed.). Boston: Little, Brown.

Ross, C. E., & Mirowsky, J. (1989). Explaining the social patterns of depression: Control and problem solving—or support and talking? *Journal of Health and Social Behavior, 30,* 206-219.

Rothbart, M. K., & Derryberry, D. (1981). Development of individual differences in temperament. In M. E. Lamb & A. L. Brown (Eds.), *Advances in developmental psychology* (Vol. I, pp. 37-86). Hillsdale, NJ: Lawrence Erlbaum.

Rothman, B. K. (1982). *Giving birth: Alternatives in childbirth.* New York: Penguin.

Santrock, J. W., & Yussen, S. R. (1992). *Child development* (5th ed.). Dubuque, IA: William C. Brown.

Schoepf, J., Bryois, C., Jonquiere, M., & Scharfetter, C. (1985). A family heredity study of postpartum "psychoses." *European Archives of Psychiatry and Neurological Sciences, 235,* 164-170.

Scott, D. (1987). Maternal and child health nurse: Role in post-partum depression. *Australian Journal of Advanced Nursing, 5,* 28-37.

Sears, W. (1991). *Christian parenting and child care* (rev. ed.). Nashville: Thomas Nelson.

Seligman, M.E.P. (1972). Learned helplessness. *Annual Review of Medicine, 23,* 407-412.

Seligman, M.E.P., & Maier, S. F. (1967). Failure to escape traumatic shock. *Journal of Experimental Psychology, 74,* 1-8.

Sgroi, S. M., & Bunk, B. S. (1988). A clinical approach to adult survivors of child sexual abuse. In S. M. Sgroi (Ed.), *Vulnerable populations* (Vol. I, pp. 137-186). Lexington, MA: Lexington Books.

Shearer, E. L. (1989). Commentary: Does cesarean delivery affect the parents? *Birth, 16,* 57-58.

Shearer, E. L., Shiono, P. H., & Rhoads, G. G. (1988). Recent trends in family-centered maternity care for cesarean birth families. *Birth, 15,* 3-7.

Shell, E. R. (1990, February). The hospital hustle. *Parenting,* pp. 57-61.

Silver, S. M. (1986). An inpatient program for post-traumatic stress disorder: Context as treatment. In C. R. Figley (Ed.), *Trauma and its wake: Vol. II. Traumatic stress theory, research, and intervention* (pp. 213-231). New York: Bruner/Mazel.

Singer, L. T., Song, L.-Y., Hill, B. P., & Jaffe, A. C. (1990). Stress and depression in mothers of failure-to-thrive children. *Journal of Pediatric Psychology, 15,* 711-720.

Skinner, E. (1991). My experience with PPP. *Heart Strings: The National Newsletter of Depression After Delivery, 2,* 1-2.

Smith, J. R. (1986). Sealing over and integration: Modes of resolution in the post-traumatic stress recovery process. In C. R. Figley (Ed.), *Trauma and its wake: Vol. II. Traumatic stress theory, research, and intervention* (pp. 20-38). New York: Bruner/Mazel.

Snaith, R. P. (1983). Pregnancy-related psychiatric disorder. *British Journal of Hospital Medicine, 29,* 450-457.

Solomon, S. D. (1986). Mobilizing social support networks in times of disaster. In C. R. Figley (Ed.), *Trauma and its wake: Vol. II. Traumatic stress theory, research, and intervention* (pp. 5-19). New York: Bruner/Mazel.

Stern, G., & Kruckman, L. (1983). Multi-disciplinary perspectives on postpartum depression: An anthropological critique. *Social Science and Medicine, 17,* 1027-1041.

Stewart, D. E. (1985). Possible relationship of postpartum psychiatric symptoms to childbirth education programmes. *Journal of Psychosomatic Obstetrics and Gynaecology, 4,* 295-301.

Susman, V. L., & Katz, J. L. (1988). Weaning and depression: Another postpartum complication. *American Journal of Psychiatry, 145,* 498-501.

Thirkettle, J. A., & Knight, R. G. (1985). The psychological precipitants of transient postpartum depression: A review. *Current Psychological Research Reviews, 4,* 143-166.

Thomas, A., & Chess, S. (1987). Commentary. In H. H. Goldsmith, A. H. Buss, R. Plomin, M. K. Rothbart, A. Thomas, S. Chess, R. R. Hinde, & R. B. McCall (Eds.), Roundtable: What is temperament? Four approaches. *Child Development, 58,* 505-529.

Tilden, V. P., & Lipson, J. G. (1981). Caesarean childbirth: Variables affecting psychological impact. *Western Journal of Nursing Research, 3,* 127-149.

Toufexis, A. (1988, June 20). Why mothers kill their babies. *Time,* pp. 81-83.

Tronick, E. Z., & Field, T. (1986). Maternal depression and infant disturbance. *New Directions for Child Development, 34,* 1-87.

Trowell, J. (1982). Possible effects of emergency caesarean section on the mother-child relationship. *Early Human Development, 7,* 41-51.

Trowell, J. (1983). Emergency caesarian section: A research study of the mother/child relationship of a group of women admitted expecting a normal vaginal delivery. *Child Abuse and Neglect, 7,* 387-394.

U.S. Advisory Board on Child Abuse and Neglect. (1991). *Creating caring communities: Blueprint for an effective federal policy on child abuse and neglect.* Washington, DC. Department of Health and Human Services.

VanderMeer, Y. G., Loendersloot, E. W., & VanLoenen, A. C. (1984). Effect of high-dose progesterone in postpartum depression. *Journal of Psychosomatic Obstetrics and Gynaecology, 3,* 67-68.

Watson, E., & Evans, S. J. (1986). An example of cross-cultural measurement of psychological symptoms in postpartum mothers. *Social Science and Medicine, 23,* 869-874.

Watson, J. P., Elliot, S. A., Rugg, A. J., & Brough, D. I. (1984). Psychiatric disorder in pregnancy and the first postnatal year. *British Journal of Psychiatry, 144,* 453-462.

Weinraub, M., & Wolf, B. (1987). Stress, social supports and parent-child interactions: Similarities and differences in single-parent and two-parent families. In C. F. Z. Boukydis (Ed.), *Research on support for parents and infants in the postnatal period* (pp. 84-113). Norwood, NJ: Ablex.

Wertz, R. W., & Wertz, D. C. (1989). *Lying in: A history of childbirth in America* (expanded ed.). New Haven, CT: Yale University Press.

Wessel, H. (1983). *Natural childbirth and the Christian family* (4th ed.). New York: Harper & Row.

Whiffen, V. E. (1988). Vulnerability to postpartum depression: A prospective multivariate study. *Journal of Abnormal Psychology, 97,* 467-474.

Whiffen, V. E., & Gotlib, I. H. (1989). Infants of postpartum depressed mothers: Temperament and cognitive status. *Journal of Abnormal Psychology, 98,* 274-279.

Wilson, J. P., & Zigelbaum, S. D. (1986). Post-traumatic stress disorder and the disposition to criminal behavior. In C. R. Figley (Ed.), *Trauma and its wake:*

Vol. II. Traumatic stress theory, research, and intervention (pp. 305-322). New York: Bruner/Mazel.

Wrate, R. M., Rooney, A. C., Thomas, P. F., & Cox, J. L. (1985). Postnatal depression and child development: A 3-year follow-up study. *British Journal of Psychiatry, 146,* 622-627.

Wurtman, R. J., & Wurtman, J. J. (1989, January). Carbohydrates and depression. *Scientific American*, pp. 68-75.

Yalom, I. D., Lunde, D. T., Moos, R. H., & Hamburg, D. A. (1968). "Postpartum blues" syndrome: A description and related variables. *Archives of General Psychiatry, 68,* 16-27.

Zborowski, M. (1969). *People in pain.* San Francisco: Jossey-Bass.

Zimbardo, P. G. (1985). *Psychology and life.* Glenview, IL: Scott, Foresman.

Author Index

Subject Index

About the Authors

Kathleen A. Kendall-Tackett is a developmental psychologist. She received her B.A. and M.A. in psychology from California State University, Chico; and her Ph.D. in developmental psychology from Brandeis University, Waltham, MA. She is currently an Assistant Research Scientist at the Stone Center at Wellesley College. This book was written while she was a Research Fellow at the Family Research Laboratory at the University of New Hampshire, Durham. Prior to receiving her Ph.D., she was Field Operations Coordinator of the Infant Health and Development Program at Stanford University's School of Medicine, Stanford, CA, and directed the Childhood Victimization Study at the Child Sexual Abuse Treatment Program in San Jose, CA. She has published articles in the fields of psychology, child abuse and neglect, and pediatrics. She is a member of the Society for Research in Child Development, the American Psychological Society, the Association for Women in Science, the American Professional Society on the Abuse of Children, and the International Society for the Prevention of Child Abuse and Neglect. She is Vice-President and a member of the Board of Directors of the Massachusetts Professional Society on the Abuse of Children. She also chairs the research committee of that organization. Her research interests include maternal depression, family violence, and high-risk infancy.

Glenda Kaufman Kantor is a nurse and sociologist/criminologist. She received her R.N. from Albert Einstein Medical Center School of Nursing in Philadelphia; her B.S. from Temple University, Philadelphia; her M.S.N. from the University of Pennsylvania, Philadelphia; and her Ph.D. in sociology from the University of Illinois. She has worked as an obstetrical and neonatal nurse, a nurse practitioner in gynecology, childbirth educator, and lactation consultant. She was an Assistant Professor of Nursing at DePaul University in Chicago and is currently a Research Associate Professor at the Family Research Laboratory at the University of New Hampshire, Durham. She was elected to Sigma Theta Tau (nursing honor society) and is a member of the American Sociological Association, the American Society of Criminologists, and the Research Society on Alcoholism. She has publications in the fields of maternal/child health, family violence, and substance abuse. Her current research interests are on the linkages between substance abuse and intrafamily violence and identifying families at risk for fatal child abuse.